Human genetic diseases

a practical approach

Human genetic diseases

a practical approach

Edited by
K E Davies

Molecular Genetics Group, Nuffield Department of Clinical
Medicine, John Radcliffe Hospital, Oxford OX3 9DU, UK

1986

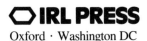
IRL PRESS
Oxford · Washington DC

IRL Press Limited,
P.O. Box 1,
Eynsham,
Oxford OX8 1JJ,
England

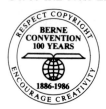
British Library Cataloguing in Publication Data

Human genetic diseases: a practical approach.
1. Medical genetics
I. Davies,K.E
616′.042   RB155

ISBN 0-947946-75-6 (softbound)
ISBN 0-947946-76-4 (hardbound)

Printed by Information Printing Ltd, Oxford, England.

Preface

DNA recombinant technology has revolutionized the antenatal diagnosis of the haemoglobinopathies in recent years. The analysis for mutations using DNA probes or oligonucleotides can be carried out after 8−10 weeks with a chorionic villi sample or at 16 weeks with amniotic fluid. This technology is now spreading so fast that many developing countries are also using this approach. The realization that restriction fragment length polymorphisms can be used as genetic markers has resulted in the demand for diagnosis of other important monogenic disorders using DNA probes. Diseases such as cystic fibrosis and Duchenne muscular dystrophy, where the biochemical defect is not yet understood, are now amenable for study if a sample is available from an affected or normal sib in the family.

This book is intended to give all the most commonly used methods for the analysis and diagnosis of human genetic diseases. The chapters cover the analysis of the DNA as well as the transcription and processing of the mRNA. Technologies that are currently being developed which will play an important role in the future, such as non-radioactive detection of DNA sequences and pulsed field electrophoresis for the separation of DNA molecules up to several thousand kilobases, are also included. The chapter on linkage analysis should be helpful for those unfamiliar with this approach for the calculation of genetic distances between DNA markers and disease loci of interest. This book should serve as a guide for anyone wishing to analyse a particular genetic disease whether for pure research purposes or for genetic counselling.

Kay Davies

Contributors

M.Antoniou
Laboratory for Gene Structure and Expression, National Institute for Medical Research, The Ridgeway, Mill Hill, London NW7 1AA, UK

V.J.Buckle
Department of Biochemistry, University of Oxford, South Parks Road, Oxford OX1 3QU, UK

I.W.Craig
Department of Biochemistry, University of Oxford, South Parks Road, Oxford OX1 3QU, UK

E.deBoer
Laboratory for Gene Structure and Expression, National Institute for Medical Research, The Ridgeway, Mill Hill, London NW7 1AA, UK

R.Fallon
Amersham International, Amersham Place, Little Chalfont, Buckinghamshire HP7 9NA, UK

H.Figueiredo
The Reynolds Building, Charing Cross and Westminster Medical School, St. Dunstan's Road, London W6 8RD, UK

F.Grosveld
Laboratory of Gene Structure and Expression, National Institute for Medical Research, The Ridgeway, Mill Hill, London NW7 1AA, UK

J.Langdale
Department of Biology, Kline Biology Tower, Yale University, New Haven, CT 06511-8112, USA

A.D.B.Malcolm
The Reynolds Building, Charing Cross and Westminster Medicial School, St. Dunstan's Road, London W6 8RD, UK

J.Old
Nuffield Department of Medicine, John Radcliffe Hospital, Oxford OX3 9DU, UK

J.Ott
Statistisches Amt der Stadt Zürich, Postfach 8022, Zürich, Switzerland

S.L.Thein
Nuffield Department of Medicine, John Radcliffe Hospital, Oxford OX3 9DU, UK

G.J.B. van Ommen
Department of Human Genetics, Wassenaarseweg 72, 2333 AL Leiden, The Netherlands

J.M.H.Verkerk
Department of Human Genetics, Wassenarrseweg 72, 2333 AL Leiden, The Netherlands

R.B.Wallace
Beckman Research Institute of the City of Hope, Department of Molecular Genetics, 1459 E.Duarte Road, Duarte, CA 91010, USA

J.L.Woodhead
The Reynolds Building, Charing Cross and Westminster Medical School, St. Dunstan's Road, London W6 8RD, UK

B.D.Young
Medical Oncology, St. Bartholomews Hospital, West Smithfield, London EC1, UK

Contents

Abbreviations

APTE	2-aminophenylthioether
BSA	bovine serum albumin
BUdR	bromodeoxyuridine
CHO	Chinese hamster ovary
DAPI	4',6-diamidino-2-phenylindole
DMD	Duchenne muscular dystrophy
DMSO	dimethylsulphoxide
DTT	dithiothreitol
EDTA	ethylemediamine tetracetic acid
EM	electron microscopy
Hepes	N-2-hydroxyethylpiperazine-N'-2-ethanesulphonic acid
HRP	horseradish peroxidase
HSR	homogeneously staining chromosomal regions
HVR	hypervariable regions
Mb	million base pairs
MOPS	3-N-morpholino-propanesulphonic acid
N/C	nitrocellulose
NP-40	Nonidet P-40
OFAGE	orthogonal field alteration gel electrophoresis
PBS	phosphate-buffered saline
PEG	polyethylene glycol
PFG	pulsed field gradient
PHA	phytohaemagglutinin
PIC	polymorphism information content
Pipes	piperazine-N,N'-bis-2-ethanesulphonic acid
PMSF	phenylmethylsulphonylfluoride
RFLP	restriction fragment length polymorphism
SSC	standard saline citrate
SDS	sodium dodecylsulphate
Tm	melting temperature
Tr	reassociation temperature

CHAPTER 1

Fetal DNA analysis

JOHN M. OLD

1. INTRODUCTION

The application of molecular biology techniques and recombinant DNA technology to the study of genetic disease has provided a wealth of information about their molecular basis at the DNA level. Perhaps the most spectacular progress has been in our understanding of the molecular defects responsible for the thalassaemia disorders and other types of haemoglobinopathies (1). This knowledge has led to the development of several methods of detecting thalassaemia and sickle cell anaemia by DNA analysis and then finally to the prenatal diagnosis of these disorders by analysis of fetal DNA obtained from amniotic-fluid cells or chorionic villi (2). These methods of DNA analysis are now being applied for the prenatal diagnosis of other important inherited diseases such as muscular dystrophy and haemophilia and it will not be long before most of the important genetic disorders can be diagnosed in an early fetus in the same way.

At present all the methods of DNA analysis for prenatal diagnosis are based on the digestion of fetal DNA with restriction endonucleases and the detection of a specific DNA fragment by hybridization of a labelled DNA probe to the digested DNA after it has been subjected to agarose gel electrophoresis and in most cases the Southern blot technique. The theory and practical details of these steps are outside the scope of this chapter and have been covered extensively in many excellent texts elsewhere (3) and also in this book. This chapter will concentrate more on the preparation and use of fetal DNA from chorionic villi and amniotic fluid cells in the different methods of DNA analysis.

2. CHORIONIC VILLI DNA

The major advance in prenatal diagnosis in recent years is the ability to obtain and utilize chorionic villi in the first trimester of pregnancy. Chorionic villi can be used for karyotyping and chromosome analysis, biochemical tests for the detection of inherited metabolic disorders, and finally as a source of DNA for gene analysis (4). The major advantage of using chorionic villi instead of amniotic fluid cells is that a diagnosis can be made in the first trimester of pregnancy which reduces the stressful period of waiting for the results and, if the fetus is affected, the couple can opt for a first trimester termination when the risks to the mother are still minimal.

2.1 Sampling procedure

Chorionic villi, which are derived from the trophoblastic layer of the developing blastocyst, can be sampled at between 8 and 12 weeks gestation. Although several different

1

sampling methods have been developed, the one most widely adopted is a single-operator aspiration technique used for an ultrasound−guided cannula (5). The villus sample should be flushed directly into a Petri dish for examination under a low-power dissecting microscope and any contaminating maternal tissue removed. If direct chromosomal preparation or cultivation of chorionic villi cells is required at a later date, the sample should be cooled from room temperature to −40°C at a rate of 1°C per minute in a tube containing a tissue culture medium supplemented with 20% fetal calf serum and 10% dimethyl sulphoxide (6). The samples are then stored in liquid nitrogen until required. If DNA analysis is required at a later date, the sample should be frozen in a tube containing a small amount of tissue culture medium in a freezer at −30°C. The frozen villi sample can then be transported safely to other laboratories for up to 48 h in dry ice.

2.2 DNA extraction procedure

The following procedure of DNA extraction is a scaled-down version of our published protocol (3) for the extraction of DNA from peripheral blood samples (*Table 1*).

(i)   Thaw the villus sample if necessary and transfer to a 1.5 ml Eppendorf tube. Spin for 5 sec in an Eppendorf centrifuge and remove the aqueous layer.

(ii)   Wash the sample by adding 0.5 ml of 150 mM NaCl, 25 mM EDTA, and mix by vortexing. Pool sample if necessary, spin and remove aqueous layer. The sample may be weighed at this stage.

(iii)   Add 0.5 ml of 150 mM NaCl, 25 mM EDTA, 5 μl of a 10% solution of SDS, 50 μg of proteinase K and mix. Incubate for 16 h at 37°C with occasional mixing to break up the sample.

(iv)   Alternatively, the villus sample may be homogenized in 0.25 ml aliquots of 150 mM NaCl, 25 mM EDTA using a 0.5 ml micro tissue homogenizer (Wheaton Scientific). Carefully pool the homogenates into a 1.5 ml Eppendorf tube and centrifuge. Remove the aqueous layer and treat the sample as in step (iii) except that only 4 h incubation at 37°C is required for complete protein digestion.

(v)   Add 0.25 ml of chloroform-isoamyl alcohol and 0.25 ml of phenol. Mix thoroughly and spin for 1 min.

(vi)   Transfer the upper aqueous layer to a clean Eppendorf tube.

(vii)   Carry out a second phenol extraction by repeating steps (v) and (vi).

(viii) Add 0.5 ml of chloroform-isoamyl alcohol, mix and spin for 1 min.

(ix)   Transfer the upper aqueous layer to a clean Eppendorf tube.

(x)   Carry out a second chloroform extraction by repeating steps (viii) and (ix).

(xi)   Precipitate the DNA (and not RNA) by adding NaCl to a final concentration of 0.4 M and two volumes of absolute ethanol at room temperature. Mix thoroughly and spin for 5 sec.

(xii)   Remove the ethanol and redissolve the DNA pellet in 50 μl of distilled water.

(xiii) Add 25 μl of 7.5 M ammonium acetate, mix and add 300 μl of absolute ethanol at room temperature. Mix and spin for 5 sec. The ammonium acetate precipitating step is included because it cleans up the DNA by solubilizing any contaminants which inhibit restriction enzymes.

(xiv)   Remove the ethanol and wash the DNA pellet with 70% ethanol. Remove the ethanol and dry the DNA pellet.

(xv)   Redissolve the DNA in 50 μl of distilled water or, if preferred, a buffer consisting of 10 mM Tris-HCl (pH 8.0), 1 mM EDTA.

(xvi)   Measure the DNA concentration of a 5 μl aliquot made up to 1 ml with distilled water. Read the absorbance at 260 nm using a 1 ml semi-micro cuvette in a double beam u.v. spectrophotometer. A DNA solution of 1 g/100 ml in a 1 cm light path has an absorbance of 200 units at 260 nm. Therefore if a reading of 0.02 is obtained, for example, this would represent a DNA concentration of 0.1 mg/100 ml or 1 μg/1 ml. Thus the 5 μl aliquot contains 1 μg of DNA and the total yield would be 10 μg (dissolved in 50 μl).

2.3 DNA yield

Chorionic villi are an excellent source of DNA and a yield of about 1 μg/mg wet weight of villus material is obtained. The size of the villus biopsy can vary enormously from as little as 5−10 mg up to 100 mg or more, and the yield of DNA varies in proportion (*Figure 1*). I have processed more than 150 villus samples for prenatal diagnosis and the average yield of DNA per sample was 35 μg. The extraction procedure described can be relied upon to isolate DNA from very small samples — in one instance only 2.5 μg of DNA was obtained. Although a result was achieved with such a small amount of DNA, whenever possible 5 μg samples of digested DNA are run routinely in my laboratory and therefore seven DNA analyses can be performed from the average-sized chorionic villus sample.

3. AMNIOTIC FLUID DNA

An alternative source of fetal DNA for prenatal diagnosis is amniotic fluid cells or cultured amniocytes. Although a second trimester diagnosis has many disadvantages com-

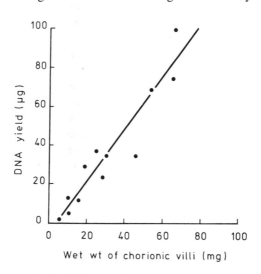

Figure 1. Graph showing the relationship between the size of chorionic villus sample and the yield of DNA.

pared with a first trimester one, this approach may be the only option for couples who present themselves too late for chorionic villus sampling or for couples who have not been previously studied by DNA analysis and an extensive family study with DNA polymorphism is required before the feasibility of prenatal diagnosis can be assessed.

3.1 Choice of sample

DNA can be prepared from amniotic fluid cells directly or from cell cultures. The disadvantage of using cultured amniocytes is that it takes $2-3$ weeks to grow amniocytes to confluency in a 25-ml flask and therefore the diagnosis is prolonged by this period. The advantage is that large amounts of fetal DNA are reliably obtained from cell cultures. Usually two or three 25-ml flasks are set up for culture and the yield of DNA from just one such flask of confluent cells is between 15 and 45 μg, enough for most purposes.

The disadvantages of preparing DNA directly from an amniotic fluid sample are that small yields of DNA are obtained and also in my limited experience of fifty amniotic fluid diagnoses, there has been a failure rate of approximately one case in ten (in which the DNA was slightly degraded and failed to produce any bands on autoradiography). The average yield of DNA from 20 ml of amniotic fluid is 7 μg which in many cases is not enough DNA to make a diagnosis (for example, at least 10 μg is required if two polymorphic markers need to be examined or if oligonucleotide probes are used). Therefore at the Oxford prenatal diagnosis laboratory, DNA is prepared from 40 ml of amniotic fluid which yields around 14 μg DNA. After sampling, the amniotic fluid sample is divided into two 25-ml Universal containers, centrifuged at 1000 g for 10 min and the amniotic fluid removed to leave just the cell pellets which are then frozen immediately to prevent degradation of the DNA.

3.2 DNA extraction procedure

The method of DNA extraction from both frozen and cultured cells is essentially identical to the method described for chorionic villi.

(i)   Thaw frozen cells in the presence of 0.5 ml of 150 mM NaCl, 25 mM EDTA and transfer them to a 1.5-ml Eppendorf tube. Centrifuge the cells and remove the supernatant. Resuspend the pellet in 0.25 ml of 150 mM NaCl, 25 mM EDTA, add 2.5 μl of 10% SDS solution and 50 μg of proteinase K. Incubate the mixture at 37°C for 4 h.

(ii)   Cultured cells are usually transported at room temperature in culture flasks topped up with tissue-culture medium. To extract DNA, decant the majority of the medium and scrape the cells off the flask surface into the remaining medium. Transfer the cells to a 50-ml plastic centrifuge tube and pellet by centrifugation at 1000 g for 10 min. Resuspend the cell pellet in 0.5 ml of 150 mM, 25 mM EDTA and treat as described above in (i).

(iii)   After proteinase K digestion, remove the protein by extracting twice with phenol-chloroform and then remove traces of phenol by two chloroform-isoamyl alcohol extractions as previously described.

(iv)   Precipitate the DNA by adding NaCl and absolute ethanol at room temperature as previously described. Occasionally, the amount of DNA present will be insufficient to precipitate as a visible mass and in these cases the ethanol mixture is placed at $-20°C$ for 1 h before centrifugation for 5 min. Both DNA and RNA will be pelleted by this procedure.

(v)   Redissolve the precipitate in distilled water (25 μl for small pellets and 50 μl for large ones). Reprecipitate the DNA by adding a half volume of 7.5 M ammonium acetate and two volumes of ethanol as previously described. The DNA concentration is now $5-10$ times greater and even very small amounts of DNA (as small as $2-3$ μg) will form a visible fibrous precipitate at room temperature. Collect the DNA by centrifugation for only 5 sec, leaving the RNA in suspension in the ethanol mixture.

(vi)   Wash the DNA pellet with 70% ethanol, dry and redissolve in 25 μl of distilled water.

(vii) Estimate the yield of DNA by measuring the absorbance of a 2.5 μl (from 25 μl) or 5 μl (from 50 μl) aliquot as previously described.

3.3 Storage of DNA

DNA solutions may be stored either at $4°C$, at $-20°C$ or at $-70°C$. The argument for storage at $4°C$ is that the DNA does not undergo repetitive freeze-thaw cycles while it is being used. Repeated freezing and thawing may shear very high molecular weight DNA (up to 100 kilobases in size) and therefore storage of DNA at $4°C$ has been recommended if the DNA is required for cloning experiments. However, in our experience, freezing and thawing does not appear to harm the DNA for the purpose of restriction endonuclease analysis. The disadvantage of storing DNA solutions at $4°C$ is that after a period of time a few samples may get ruined by microbial growth unless an antimicrobial agent is added.

In our laboratory, DNA samples are stored at $-20°C$ in 1.5 ml Eppendorf tubes in a sectioned aluminium tray storage system designed by Denly Instruments Ltd to fit a domestic upright freezer. In our experience, this is a more convenient storage system than a similar set up in a $-70°C$ freezer and the DNA samples have been kept for up to four years at $-20°C$ without any apparent deterioration. However, it has been proposed that at this temperature micro-pockets of non-frozen liquid of high salt concentration may exist which could promote the disruption of DNA. Storage at $-70°C$ would remove this problem.

Table 1. Preparation of DNA from 20 ml blood.

---

1.   Fresh blood must be collected in tubes containing the anticoagulants EDTA or heparin, otherwise the sample will clot and provide very little DNA. The sample may be kept at $-4°C$ for several days without deterioration, or frozen and kept indefinitely at $-70°C$ or up to six months at $-20°C$.
2.   Add 30 ml of distilled water to fresh or thawed sample, mix and centrifuge at 3000 g for 10 min. Remove the supernatant.
3.   Add 25 ml of 0.1% Nonidet P40 solution to the pellet, mix and spin.
4.   Add 10 ml of 100 mM NaCl, 25 mM EDTA to the pellet and mix.
5.   Add 0.5 mg of proteinase K, 0.5 ml of 10% SDS, and incubate at $37°C$ for $4-16$ h.
6.   Carry out two phenol-chloroform extractions (5 ml of each).
7.   Carry out two chloroform extractions.
8.   Precipitate the DNA at room temperature by adding 1 ml of 4 M NaCl and 22 ml of absolute ethanol.
9.   Redissolve the DNA in 1 ml of either distilled water or in 10 mM Tris-HCl (pH 7.5), 1 mM EDTA overnight at $+4°C$.
10. Measure the DNA concentration.

---

4. DNA ANALYSIS

The fundamental principle on which most methods of DNA analysis are based is the molecular hybridization of a small amount of pure labelled DNA probe to a much larger amount of genomic DNA. The probe and target DNA are first denatured to make them single-stranded and then under the right experimental conditions they are allowed to reassociate with one another to form double-stranded labelled molecules. Under the right experimental conditions the probe only hybridizes to a perfectly-matching genomic DNA sequence, i.e. its complementary sequence and the unhybridized and mismatched probe is removed by washing. The remaining probe – genomic DNA hybrids are identified by autoradiography if the probes are labelled with [^{32}P]dCTP, or by staining if a non-radioactive label such as biotin is used.

An outline of the procedure currently used in our laboratory is listed in *Tables 2* and *3*. The first step is to cleave a sample of genomic DNA (usually 5 or 10 μg) with an appropriate restriction endonuclease. The digested DNA is then loaded into a well of an agarose gel and subjected to electrophoresis. The DNA fragments are negatively charged and migrate towards the anode according to their size. After running the gel for sufficient time to separate the fragments, the gel is stained with ethidium bromide and photographed under u.v. illumination to provide a visual record. The gel is then soaked in alkali to denature the DNA, neutralized and set up for transfer of the fragments onto a nitrocellulose or nylon filter by the method known as Southern blotting, as shown in *Figure 2*.

Nitrocellulose is now being replaced in many laboratories by nylon filters such as Hybond N (Amersham) as it is much stronger and can be reprobed many times. For DNA analysis with oligonucleotide probes, the gel may be dried down after the neutralization step and the probe hybridized to the DNA in the dried gel instead. After blotting the DNA is fixed to the filter by baking (nitrocellulose or nylon) or by u.v. irradiation (nylon only) and then hybridized to a specific probe labelled by nick translation or hexanucleotide priming. The hybridization is usually carried out in a polythene bag made by heat sealing two sheets of polythene sandwiching the filter. After a short pre-soak period, the labelled probe is added to the bag and the filter hybridized either at 65°C

Table 2. Restriction enzyme digestion of DNA.

1. Digest 5 μg of DNA with 10 units of enzyme under the manufacturer's conditions in a volume of 30 μl. The incubation is carried out for at least 4 h and extra enzyme may be added at the halfway stage. The presence of spermidine trihydrochloride (pH 7.0, 1 – 5 mM) may help to overcome any enzyme inhibitors in the DNA sample.
2. If the DNA fails to digest, reprecipitate a small aliquot of the DNA with ammonium acetate or spermine as described below and repeat with fresh enzyme.
    (i) Ammonium acetate method. Add half volume of 7.5 M ammonium acetate and 2 volumes of absolute ethanol. Spin and wash the precipitate with 70% ethanol. Dry, redissolve and measure the concentration.
    (ii) Spermine precipitation method (does not work so well for large amounts of DNA). Add spermine solution (100 mM) to give a final concentration of 3 mM, mix and spin. Redissolve the precipitate in a small volume of 0.5 M NaCl (large amounts of DNA are difficult to dissolve). Add two volumes of ethanol and carry on as in ammonium acetate method (i).
3. Add 5 μg of bromophenol blue/Ficoll solution and mix.

Table 3. A method of Southern blotting.

1. Load the sample into a well of a horizontal agarose gel (usually 0.8% in TBE[a] or AGB[a]) and run submerged in buffer for 16 h at approximately 1.5 V/cm.
2. Stain the gel by immersion in ethidium bromide solution (1 mg/l) for 5 min and photograph under u.v. light.
3. Soak the gel in 1 M NaOH for 1 h.
4. Neutralize the gel in 1 M Tris-HCl (pH 7.5), 3 M NaCl for 3 h.
5. Set up Southern blot as shown in *Figure 2* for an overnight transfer of DNA to a nitrocellulose or nylon filter with 6 × SSC.
6. Bake the filter for 2 h at 80°C under vacuum.
7. Pre-soak the filter in polythene bag containing 5−10 ml of pre-soak buffer[a] at 42°C for 1 h.
8. Label the DNA probes with [^{32}P]dCTP (PB10205, Amersham) with a nick-translation kit (N50000, Amersham) or a hexanucleotide primer kit (polymeroid RH, P and S Biochemicals).
9. Squeeze out the pre-soak buffer and add approximtely 25 ng of ^{32}P-labelled probe (10−30 × 10^6 c.p.m.) in 1−2 ml of hybridization buffer[a]. Reseal and incubate at 42°C for 16 h.
10. Remove the filter and wash it three times with 500 ml of 2 × SSC at room temperature.
11. Wash the filter twice at 65°C with 0.1 × SSC/0.1% SDS in a shaking water bath. NB: Such conditions may be too stringent for some probes (e.g. the X-chromosome specific 'pERT' probes need to be hot-washed in 3 × SSC).
12. Dry or wrap the filters in cling film and autoradiograph in cassettes with intensifying screens at −80°C for 16 h if fast film (e.g. Kodak XAR-5) is used or for 1−3 days if cheaper ordinary X-ray film is used (e.g. Fuji RX).

NB: The alkali blotting method (see text) is now working well in our laboratory. Omit step (4), blot onto Hybond N (Amersham) overnight with 1 M NaOH as transfer buffer, wash the filter in 2 × SSC after blotting and dry. Step (6) is then omitted.

[a]For composition of TBE, AGB, pre-soak and hybridization buffers, see *Table 4*.

Table 4. Stock solutions mentioned in protocols.

500 mM EDTA	Add 18.6 g of EDTA to 100 ml of distilled water. Adjust pH to 7.5 by adding NaOH pellets until EDTA just dissolves.
Chloroform-isoamyl alcohol (25:1)	Add 100 ml of isoamyl alcohol to 1.5 l of chloroform.
Phenol (ultrapure or redistilled grade)	Dissolve 1.5 kg in 165 ml of distilled water. Add 200 ml of 1 M Tris-HCl (pH 8.0), mix and remove aqueous layer. Repeat twice. Add 8-hydroxyquinoline to a final concentration of 0.1%. Add an equal volume of 0.1 M Tris-HCl (pH 8.0), 0.2% β-mercaptoethanol and remove the aqueous layer.
Ficoll/bromophenol blue	15% Ficoll 400/0.05% bromophenol blue in 1 × AGB.
TBE	89 mM Tris-HCl, 89 mM boric acid, 2.5 mM EDTA. Do not adjust pH. Make up 10 ×.
AGB	40 mM Tris-HCl, 20 mM sodium acetate, 0.2 mM EDTA. Adjust pH to 8.3 with acetic acid. Usually made up as 50 ×.
SSC	0.15 mM NaCl, 0.015 M sodium citrate. Usually made up as 20 ×.
Pre-soak buffer	50% formamide, 3 × SSC, 10 × Denhardt's, 20 μg/ml sonicated denatured salmon sperm DNA (SS DNA), 2% SDS.
Hybridization buffer	50% formamide, 3 × SSC, 1 × Denhardt's, 20 μg/ml SS DNA, 10 μg poly(A)/10% dextran sulphate, 2% SDS.
Denhardt's	0.02% Ficoll 400, 0.02% BSA, 0.02% polyvinylpyrrolidene.

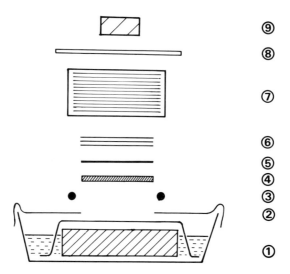

Figure 2. Cross section of a Southern blot apparatus. The components are: (**1**) tray containing 6 × SSC and a slab of saturated foam sponge covered with a sheet of thick filter paper; (**2**) cling film cover surrounding the gel; (**3**) support for towels, e.g. a 10 ml pipette; (**4**) agarose gel; (**5**) nitrocellulose or nylon filter; (**6**) several sheets of filter paper (gel size); (**7**) stack of paper towels; (**8**) glass sheet; (**9**) weight.

or at 42°C if 50% formamide is included in the hybridization mixture. The filter is washed under conditions appropriate for the particular probe and subjected to auto-radiography (if radioactive).

The basic technique of restriction endonuclease analysis was introduced in 1975 by Southern (7) and most laboratories have since developed and modified the method to suit the requirements of the investigators. The method used in my laboratory for the detection of the haemoglobinopathies has been published in complete detail elsewhere and the method for oligonucleotide analysis is described in another chapter in this book. Many laboratory manuals have also been published which cover this technique, the best is probably the one written by T.Maniatis and co-workers (8).

4.1 Direct detection

At present there are three different approaches to the direct direction of a genetic disorder by DNA analysis: (a) the direct hybridization of a gene-specific probe, (b) the use of a mutation-specific restriction endonuclease, (c) the use of oligonucleotide probes to detect a point mutation. The main advantages of a direct analysis are that all at-risk fetuses can be diagnosed and that the time-consuming pedigree studies required for linkage analysis of restriction fragment length polymorphism (RFLP) are not necessary, although both parents still have to be studied to identify their molecular defect and confirm their heterozygosity. DNA from normal and affected individuals are also usually run simultaneously as controls.

Gene-specific probes can be used directly to detect a recessive genetic disorder if it results from a deletion of part or all of the genomic DNA sequence complementary to the DNA probe. If part of the probe sequence is deleted, the probe will hybridize to a different restriction fragment to the one generated from the normal chromosome

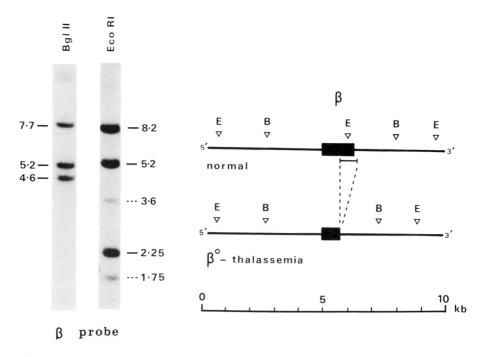

Figure 3. Direct detection of a deletion type of β°-thalassaemia. The location of the *Bgl*II sites (B) and *Eco*RI sites (E) at the normal β-globin gene locus is shown, together with a map of the β°-thalassaemia gene which results from a 619 base pair deletion at the 3' end of the β-globin gene. An autoradiograph shows the various *Bgl*II and *Eco*RI fragments detected with a β-globin gene probe. The β°-thalassaemia gene produces a smaller abnormal 4.6 kb *Bgl*II fragment and a larger 8.2 kb *Eco*RI fragment (due to the loss of an *Eco*RI site). The 7.7, 2.25 and 1.76 kb fragments contain cross-hybridizing δ-globin gene fragments.

and thus the homozygous condition for the genetic disorder is diagnosed by the presence of the characteristic abnormal fragment and the absence of the normal one. $\delta\beta$-Thalassaemia, Hb Lepore, and one type of β°-thalassaemia (*Figure 3*) are due to DNA deletions (9) and can be diagnosed this way. If the whole of the probe sequence is deleted, the homozygous condition is characterized by the complete absence of any DNA fragments which hybridize to the probe. Certain types of α-thalassaemia (10) can be detected in this way with an α-globin probe (as shown in *Figure 4*). Such disorders may also be detected by a simple dot-blot or slot-blot method in which the DNA fragments are not subjected to electrophoresis but simply dotted onto a filter before hybridization to the probe (11). For genetic disorders located on the X chromosome the absence of hybridization of a specific probe may be used to detect a gene deletion in males. However, the identification of females with a deletion is technically more difficult as it depends on detecting only half the hybridization signal compared with that generated by an equal amount of normal female DNA and is usually achieved by measuring the density of the bands on the autoradiograph.

The second method, the use of a mutation-specific restriction endonuclease, can only be used when the molecular defect responsible for the disorder abolishes or creates a new restriction enzyme recognition site. The best example of such a disorder is sickle-cell anaemia, in which a single base change of A to T in codon 6 of the β-globin gene

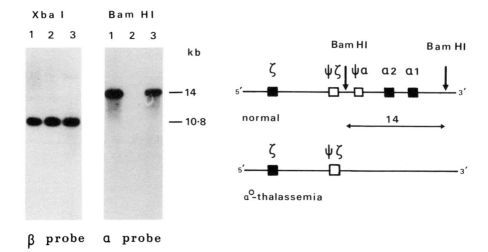

Figure 4. Direct detection of a complete gene deletion. A map of the normal α-globin gene locus is shown, together with a map of the DNA deletion which removes both α-globin genes and results in the phenotype of α°-thalassaemia. An autoradiograph shows the detection of the homozygous condition for α°-thalassaemia by the absence of a 14 kb *Bam*HI fragment (track 2). Track 1 contains normal DNA, and track 3 contains DNA from an α°-thalassaemic heterozygote. All three DNAs hybridize to a β-globin gene probe when digested with *Xba*I.

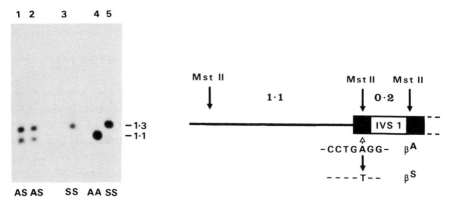

Figure 5. Direct detection of sickle-cell anaemia by using a mutation-specific restriction endonuclease. A map of the 5' end of the β-globin gene shows the location of the sickle cell point mutation and the recognition sites of *Mst*II, one of which is abolished by the sickle cell mutation. The autoradiograph shows a prenatal diagnosis using *Mst*II digested DNA hybridized to a β-globin gene probe. Tracks 1 and 2 contain DNA from the parents (both sickle cell trait, genotype AS), track 3 contains fetal DNA, and tracks 4 and 5 contain normal (AA) and homozygous sickle cell DNA (SS) controls.

destroys a site for the enzyme *Mst*II (12). An example of a prenatal diagnosis of sickle-cell anaemia by *Mst*II analysis is shown in *Figure 5*.

Sickle-cell anaemia can also be detected by a third direct approach, oligonucleotide hybridization (13). This method, described in detail in another chapter, is used for the detection of disorders resulting from a single base mutation. To date it has been used for the diagnosis of several types of β-thalassaemia (14) and for α_1-antitrypsin deficiency (15).

genotypes

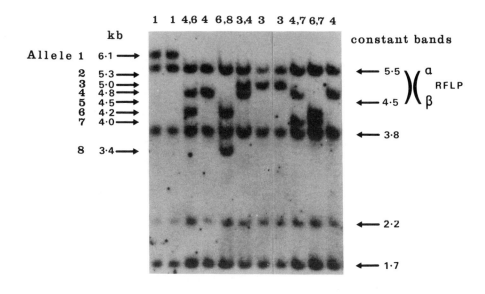

Figure 6. Autoradiograph showing the hypervariable DNA polymorphism detected with the X-chromosome specific probe St14. The sizes of eight common alleles are shown on the left of the autoradiograph and the alleles present in 11 individuals are indicated at the top. The St14 probe also hybridizes to three constant *Taq*I fragments and detects a simple RFLP labelled α and β. No β allele is present in the 11 DNA samples shown here.

4.2 Indirect detection

Naturally occurring variations in DNA sequence can be detected by restriction endonuclease analysis. These RFLPs can be used in informative families for prenatal diagnosis by analysis of their linkage to the mutant gene. The most useful RFLPs are the highly variable regions of DNA composed of tandemly repeated short DNA sequences. One such highly polymorphic region close to the α-globin gene locus (16) has recently been shown to be linked to the gene responsible for polycystic kidney disease (17). Because of the large number of polymorphic fragments from one locus, most individuals will usually have two differently sized fragments and therefore such loci are extremely useful as genetic markers. For example, *Figure 6* shows a highly variable DNA polymorphism that is closely linked to haemophilia A and can be used in more than 90% of families at risk for this disorder (18). However, highly variable DNA regions have not been located near most genetic disorders and therefore in most cases ordinary RFLPs have to be used as markers. These occur if a variation in DNA sequence creates a new restriction enzyme site or abolishes an existing one. This type of polymorphism has only two forms, usually denoted + if the enzyme site is present and − if the site is absent. The polymorphic DNA fragments are inherited in a simple Mendelian fashion and can be used as genetic markers for prenatal diagnosis. An example of such a polymorphism is shown in *Figure 7* which illustrates a prenatal diagnosis of haemophilia A using a *Bgl*II polymorphism detected with the probe DX13 which is also closely linked to the factor VIII gene locus (19).

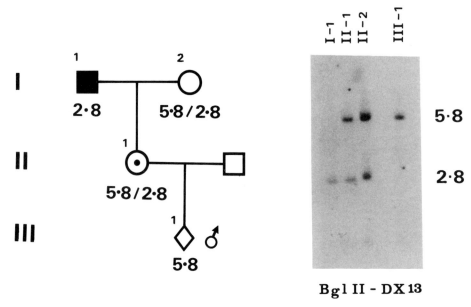

Bgl II - DX 13

Figure 7. Prenatal diagnosis of haemophilia A by linkage analysis by a *Bgl*II restriction fragment length polymorphism detected by the X-chromosome specific probe DX13. An autoradiograph shows the distribution of the two polymorphic fragments of 5.8 and 2.8 kb in three family members and the fetal DNA sample (III.1). In the pedigree, an affected male is represented by the shaded square, a normal female by the open circle, a carrier female by the inclusion of a spot and the fetus by a diamond symbol. The fetus was shown to be male by karyotyping and a 92% chance of being normal by linkage analysis (DX13 is approximately 8 centimorgans from the haemophilia A locus).

There are many disadvantages in using RFLPs for prenatal diagnosis instead of one of the direct methods. The most important ones are the potential for recombination between the disease gene and the polymorphic site and the difficulty in obtaining informative siblings or relatives for pedigree analysis. To be useful, a polymorphic marker must be closely linked to the site of the disease mutation. For several disorders, such as Huntington's chorea and Duchenne muscular dystrophy, the location and nature of molecular defects are unknown and the RFLPs available are all five or more centimorgans (one centimorgan is very approximately one thousand kilobase pairs) from the disease gene (20,21). Consequently such markers are only of limited use on their own. The use of two RFLPs, one on either side of the disease gene, overcomes this problem to a certain extent although the probability of an individual having two polymorphic flanking markers is usually quite low. Finally, even when the RFLPs are only a few kilobase pairs away from the disease gene the chance of recombination may still be quite high if a hotspot for DNA recombination is located between the markers and the mutation. Such a hotspot exists inside the β-globin gene clusters (22) and at least one crossover has been reported (23) between a β-thalassaemia mutation and a polymorphic restriction site only 15 kilobase pairs apart.

The majority of RFLPs do not exist in linkage disequilibrium with genetic disorders and therefore when an individual is found to be informative for an RFLP, a further study of DNA from other members of the family is required in order to assign the phase of the RFLP. Although it is often difficult to obtain DNA from key family members for a variety of reasons, the RFLP linkage method is more applicable than the direct methods as it can be used for any genetic disorder independent of whether the molecular defect has been determined. At the moment, RFLPs may be used to diagnose β-thalassaemia, haemophilia A, phenylketonuria, ornithine transcarbamylase deficiency, antithrombin-3 deficiency, polycystic kidney disease, Huntington's chorea and Duchenne muscular dystrophy (24); in the immediate future, for cystic fibrosis, for which closely linked DNA probes have just recently been found (25−27).

5. POTENTIAL PROBLEMS OF DNA ANALYSIS

Fetal diagnoses by DNA analysis have many potential pitfalls, including (a) maternal contamination, (b) DNA probe contamination of DNA samples, (c) technical difficulties with the Southern blotting methodology, and (d) non-paternity.

5.1 **Maternal contamination**

Chorionic villus biposies are usually contaminated with maternal decidua which can be easily identified under a low-power microscope and removed. As diagnoses by DNA analysis are usually performed with DNA from uncultured villi, a small amount of maternal decidua remaining in the sample should not affect the diagnosis as any autoradiograph bands from a small percentage of maternal DNA will be very weak compared with the fetal DNA band. Maternal DNA contamination may be monitored by hybridizing a highly polymorphic DNA probe for a variable DNA region because the mother is usually heterozygous for such a polymorphism and often has different polymorphic bands to the father. The presence of only one maternal polymorphic restriction fragment in the fetal DNA could indicate the absence of any contaminating maternal DNA. An attempt at such a study with a highly polymorphic X-chromosome specific probe has been reported by Elles *et al.* (28) who observed no maternal contamination after exposure of the autoradiograph for 7 days and concluded that any DNA present was less than 2% of the total DNA.

5.2 **Plasmid contamination**

Contamination of DNA samples or stock solutions with plasmid DNA has been reported to have caused at least two misdiagnoses. Plasmid contamination is a problem which is encountered from time to time in most laboratories in which plasmid probes are grown up and prepared in the same working area as DNA samples are processed. This problem is identified by the presence of strange bands on the autoradiograph which are often so strong as to obscure the weaker-hybridizing genomic DNA fragments (*Figure 8*). Rewashing the filter and rehybridizing it with a pure genomic DNA fragment probe can often solve this problem, although tracing the source of the contamination has, in our experience, often proved unsuccessful and the only remedy is to remake every suspect stock solution from its basic ingredients.

5.3 **Technical difficulties**

Both the direct and indirect methods of DNA analysis occasionally suffer from various technical difficulties. One important problem because of the small quantities of DNA obtained from chorionic villi and amniotic fluid samples is the incomplete (partial) diges-

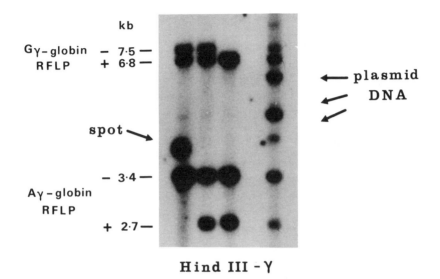

Figure 8. Autoradiograph illustrating two technical problems of DNA analysis. Four DNA samples digested with *Hind*III and hybridized to a γ-globin gene probe illustrate the various polymorphic fragments generated by a *Hind*III site in both the ^{G}γ-globin gene and the ^{A}γ-globin gene. Track 4 also contains three strongly hybridizing bands due to plasmid contamination. A second problem is also illustrated — the presence of random spots of radioactivity, one of which in track 1 is larger than the signal produced by the bands themselves.

tion of DNA by restriction enzymes. Often only enough DNA is obtained for one attempt at a diagnosis and a partial digestion of the DNA sample, which results in a multiple band pattern as shown in *Figure 9*, is often uninterpretable with respect to making a diagnosis. Partial digestions are caused by either the loss of activity of the restriction enzyme or the presence of an enzyme inhibitor in the DNA preparation. The latter can be overcome by purifying the DNA by ammonium acetate precipitation (as described in the protocol for chorionic villi DNA preparation) or by spermine precipitation (29), and also by adding spermidine (30) to the restriction enzyme buffer (at a final concentration of 1−4 mM) as described in *Table 2*.

Another problem which is often encountered with the Southern blotting technique is a poor transfer of DNA from the gel to the filter. High molecular weight fragments transfer very inefficiently and the transfer may be improved by breaking up the fragments before transfer either by soaking the gel in 0.25 M HCl for 15 min or by prolonged exposure to u.v. radiation. Non-transfer of fragments could lead to problems with a diagnosis for a gene-deletion disorder and thus appropriate control DNAs should be run alongside the fetal sample and also a second gene probe included in the hybridization mixture which hybridizes to an unrelated sequence in the fetal DNA in a similar size range as the diagnostic fragment.

6. FUTURE DEVELOPMENTS

Fetal diagnosis by analysis of chorionic villi DNA is rapidly becoming an established technique as more obstetricians worldwide are gaining expertise in the sampling procedure. However, an unanswered question at the moment is the safety of the procedure

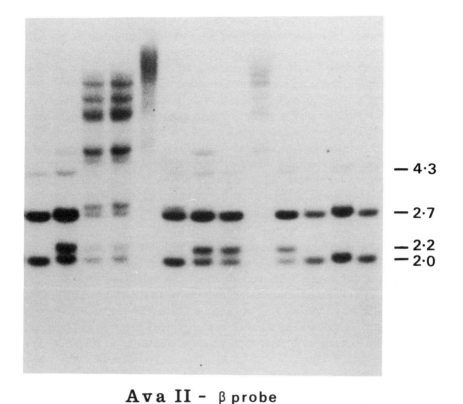

Ava II - β probe

Figure 9. Autoradiograph showing examples of partially and undigested DNA. DNA samples were digested with *Ava*II and hybridized to a β-globin gene probe. Two constant bands of 4.3 and 2.7 kb are detected in addition to two polymorphic bands of 2.0 and 2.2 kb. Tracks 3, 4 and 9 contain partially digested DNA, and track 5 undigested DNA.

to the fetus. Over 4000 chorionic villus samplings have now been performed worldwide for which an overall fetal loss rate of 4.1% has been reported (31). Once the natural incidence of spontaneous abortion in the first trimester of pregnancy has been accurately determined and taken into account, the risks to the fetus will probably prove to be not much higher than that for amniocentesis and first trimester fetal diagnosis will become widely accepted.

Although chorionic villi are a good source of DNA, occasionally very small samples are obtained and therefore the ability to carry out a diagnosis on 1 μg or less of DNA would be a major improvement. This could be achieved by increasing the specific activity of the probes by using a non-radioactive labelling technique or by improving the efficiency of the Southern blot method. At present, non-radioactively labelled probes, such as biotin-labelled, are less sensitive than radioactive ones by about a factor of ten, but many companies are working on this problem and the methodology could develop very fast to a point where it is better than ^{32}P-labelling. Many ideas have been suggested in the past to improve the Southern blotting method without much effect but the introduction of nylon filters seems to be a significant advance. It has recently been reported that DNA fragments can be blotted onto nylon filters straight after being denatured with alkali (32). This modification removes the requirement for gel neutralization and the opportunity for the DNA fragments to diffuse in the gel. Blotting in alkali also fixes the DNA to the filter, removing the need for baking or exposure to u.v. light. According to the report, this modification results in sharper bands and the detection of single copy sequences in less than 1 μg of genomic DNA.

Improvements in the sensitivity of the Southern blotting technique such as this will lead to the use of smaller gels and a much simpler procedure which should be able to be automated and packaged as a diagnostic kit. Such a development, coupled with a sensitive non-radioactive labelling method to generate DNA probes which can be kept indefinitely, will enable the technique to be applied outside of the specialized laboratory and result in a much wider application in the diagnosis of genetic disorders.

7. DNA ANALYSIS – RECENT IMPROVEMENTS

Since the writing of this chapter, an important improvement in the sensitivity of prenatal diagnosis tests using DNA probes has been reported. This method involves the amplification of the sequence of interest before hybridization to the radioactive or non-radioactive probe (33). This technique has enabled the detection of sickle cell anaemia in samples containing significantly less than 1 μg of genomic DNA. This method will be helpful in the tests where oligonucleotides are used as probes (see Chapter 3) and in the detection of base-pair mismatches by electrophoresis under denaturing conditions (34).

8. REFERENCES

1. Collins,F.S. and Weissman,S.M. (1984) *Prog. Nucleic Acid Res. Mol. Biol.*, **31**, 315.
2. Old,J.M. (1986) in *Genetic Disorders of the Fetus*, Milunsky,A. (ed.), Plenum Publishing Corporation, New York, in press.
3. Old,J.M. and Higgs,D.R. (1983) in *Methods in Hematology*, Weatherall,D.J. (ed.), Churchill Livingstone, Edinburgh, Vol. 6, p. 74.
4. Rodeck,C.H. (1984) in *Prenatal Diagnosis*, Rodeck,C.H. and Nicolaides,K.H. (eds), Royal College of Obstetricians and Gynaecologists, London, p. 15.
5. Rodeck,C.H., Morsman,J.M., Nicolaides,K.H., McKenzie,C., Gosden,C.M. and Gosden,J.R. (1983) *Lancet*, **ii**, 1340.
6. Endres,M., Dawson,G., Wirtz,A. and Haaindl,E. (1985) in *First Trimester Fetal Diagnosis*, Fraccaro,M., Simoni,G. and Brambati,B. (eds), Springer-Verlag, Berlin, p. 201.
7. Southern,E.M. (1975) *J. Mol. Biol.*, **98**, 503.
8. Maniatis,T., Fritsch,E.F. and Sambrook,J. (1982) *Molecular Cloning. A Laboratory Manual*, Cold Spring Harbor Laboratory Press, New York.
9. Weatherall,D.J. and Clegg,J.B. (1981) *The Thalassaemia Syndromes*, 3rd edition, Blackwell Scientific Publications, Oxford.
10. Higgs,D.R. and Weatherall,D.J. (1983) in *Current Topics in Haematology*, Piomelli,S. and Yachin,S. (eds), Alan R.Liss, New York, Vol. 4, p. 37.
10. Rubin,E.M. and Kan,Y.W. (1985) *Lancet*, **i**, 75.
12. Orkin,S.H., Little,P.F.R., Kazazian,H.H. and Boehm,C.D. (1982) *New Engl. J. Med.*, **307**, 32.
13. Connor,B.J., Reyes,A.A., Morin,C., Itakura,K., Teplitz,R.L. and Wallace,R.B. (1983) *Proc. Natl. Acad. Sci. USA*, **80**, 278.
14. Weatherall,D.J., Old,J.M., Thein,S.L., Wainscoat,J.S. and Clegg,J.B. (1985) *J. Med. Genet.*, **22**, 422.
15. Kidd,J.V., Wallace,R.B., Itakura,K. and Woo,S.L. (1983) *Nature*, **304**, 230.
16. Higgs,D.R., Goodbourn,S.E.Y., Wainscoat,J.S., Clegg,J.B. and Weatherall,D.J. (1981) *Nucleic Acids Res.*, **9**, 4213.
17. Reeders,S.T., Breuning,M.H., Davies,K.E., Nicholls,R.D., Jarman,A.P., Higgs,D.R., Pearson,P.L. and Weatherall,D.J. (1985) *Nature*, **317**, 542.
18. Oberle,I., Camerino,G., Heilig,R., Grunebaum,L., Cazenave,J.-P., Crapanzano,C., Mannucci,P.M. and Mandel,J.-L. (1985) *New Engl. J. Med.*, **312**, 682.

19. Harper,K., Winter,R.M., Pembrey,M.E., Hartley,D., Davies,K.E. and Tuddenham,E.G.D. (1984) *Lancet*, **ii**, 6.
20. Gusella,J.F., Wexler,M.S., Conneally,P.M., Naylor,S.L., Anderson,M.A., Tanzi,R.E., Watkins,P.C., Ottina,K., Wallace,M.R., Sakaguchi,A.Y., Young,A.B., Shoulson,I., Bonilla,E. and Martin,J.B. (1983) *Nature*, **306**, 234.
21. Drayna,D. and White,R. (1985) *Science*, **230**, 753.
22. Chakravarti,A., Buetow,K.H., Antonarakis,S.E., Waber,P.G., Boehm,C.D. and Kazazian,H.H. (1984) *Am. J. Human Genet.*, **36**, 1239.
23. Old,J.M., Heath,C., Fitches,A., Thein,S.L., Jeffreys,A.J., Petrou,M., Modell,B. and Weatherall,D.J. (1986) *J. Med. Genet.*, in press.
24. Old,J.M. and Davies,K.E. (1986) in *Biosensors*, Turner,A.P.F., Karube,I. and Wilson,G.S. (eds), Oxford University Press, in press.
25. Knowlton,R.G., Cohen-Haguenauer,O., Van Cong,N., Frezal,J., Brown,V.A., Borker,D., Braman,J.C., Schumm,J.W., Tsui,L-C., Buchwald,M. and Davis-Keller,H. (1985) *Nature*, **318**, 380.
26. White,R., Woodward,S., Leppert,M., O'Connell,P., Hoff,M., Herbst,J., Lalouel,J.-M., Dean,M. and Woude,G.V. (1985) *Nature*, **318**, 392.
27. Wainright,B.J., Scambler,P.J., Schmidtke,E., Watson,E.A., Law,H.-Y., Farrall,M., Cooke,C.J., Eiberg,H. and Williamson,R. (1985) *Nature*, **318**, 384.
28. Elles,R.B., Williamson,R., Niazi,M., Coleman,D.V. and Horwell,D. (1983) *New Engl. J. Med.*, **308**, 1433.
29. Hoopes,B.C. and McClare,W.R. (1981) *Nucleic Acids Res.*, **9**, 5493.
30. Bouche,J.P. (1981) *Anal. Biochem.*, **115**, 42.
31. Jackson,Z. (1985) in *Chorionic Villi Sampling Newsletter*, Jefferson Medical College, Thomas Jefferson University, Philadelphia.
32. Reed,K.C. and Mann,D.A. (1985) *Nucleic Acid Res.*, **20**, 7207.
33. Saiki, R.K., Scharf, S., Faloona, F., Mullis, K.B., Horn, G.T., Erlich, H.A. and Arnheim, N. (1985) *Science*, **230**, 1350.
34. Myers, R.M., Lumelsky,N., Lerman,L.S. and Maniatis,T. (1985) *Nature*, **313**, 495.

CHAPTER 2

A short guide to linkage analysis

JURG OTT

1. INTRODUCTION

This contribution serves two purposes. First, it should be a simple introduction to the analysis of human genetic linkage for the novice who has not been exposed to this field at all, and secondly, for individuals with experience, it gives a summary of the steps involved in a linkage analysis and presents a few new findings and particular twists in linkage analysis.

Short discussions of linkage analysis may be found in most human genetics texts. A more detailed representation is that of Conneally and Rivas (1). For a comprehensive treatment of linkage analysis, the reader is referred to my book on linkage analysis (2) that also provides an introduction to the basic genetic terms not given here.

Consider two gene loci. As is well known in genetics, each individual carries two alleles at each locus and, with probability one half, transmits one of the two alleles from each locus to an offspring. Generally, the four possible selections (gametes) of two non-allelic genes, one from each of the two loci, are transmitted in an approximate 1:1:1:1 ratio. For specific pairs of loci, however, one observes a deviation from this ratio in the sense that the two non-allelic genes received from one parent of an individual tend to be transmitted together to the offspring of this individual. This phenomenon is called *genetic linkage*, and loci showing genetic linkage are termed *genetically linked*.

Usually, genetic linkage is not complete so that even for linked loci, non-allelic genes received from two parents recombine such that an individual may transmit to an offspring one gene at one locus received from the mother and one gene at another, linked locus received from the father. Therefore, it is not usually meaningful to speak of linked *alleles* but only of linked loci. The proportion of such recombinations out of all opportunities for recombination (recombinations and non-recombinations) is called the *recombination fraction*, denoted by the Greek letter θ (theta). For unlinked gene loci, according to the 1:1:1:1 ratio mentioned above, the recombination fraction is equal to 50%, while for linked loci it is less than 50%. Based on determinations of the recombination fraction in the fruitfly, early geneticists have been able to determine that all gene loci of that fly can be grouped into a certain rather small number of linkage groups where one linkage group comprises all those loci that are genetically linked to at least one other locus in the group. Except for a different number of linkage groups in different organisms, genetic linkage and linkage groups could be shown to exist in most plants and animals including man.

The cytological equivalent of a linkage group is the chromosome and the gene loci on it. It turns out that loci far apart on the same chromosome, or located on different

$\hat{\theta}$, of the recombination fraction. This intuitively appealing estimation method goes back to the distinguished statistician R.A.Fisher and can be shown to extract all the information contained on θ in the observations. It affords an elegant way to deal with missing and partially missing information (6).

In linkage analysis, it is not so much the value of $L(\theta)$ that is of interest but rather the ratio, $L(\theta)/L(0.5)$, called *odds ratio* or *odds for linkage*. As it is somewhat inconvenient to work with likelihoods or odds ratios, it has become customary in linkage analysis to use the decimal logarithm of the odds ratio, the so-called *lod* or *lod score*,

$$Z(\theta) - \log_{10}[L(\theta)/L(0.5)]$$

In the estimation of the recombination fraction, one calculates $Z(\theta)$ for the sequence of θ values, $\theta = 0, 0.001, 0.05, 0.1, 0.2, 0.3$ and 0.4 (standard lod table, 7), and picks that value of θ as the most plausible value at which $Z(\theta)$ is largest. In simple situations, $Z(\theta)$ may be derived by hand from first principles but usually $Z(\theta)$ has to be calculated numerically with the aid of a computer program (see Section 5). 'Negative' evidence for linkage is obtained when $Z(\theta)$ is highest at $\theta = 0.5$. Then, by construction, $Z(\theta) = 0$. If a certain body of data is completely uninformative for linkage, then $Z(\theta)$ will be equal to zero for all values of θ. In the simple example of one recombinant and three non-recombinants, $Z(\theta) = \log[\theta(1-\theta)^3/0.0625]$ with a maximum of $Z = 0.227$ at $\hat{\theta} = 0.25$. The odds for linkage are then $0.25(0.75)^3/0.0625$ or about $1.7:1$.

Sometimes, in a linkage analysis one can simply count recombinants and non-recombinants in which case the observed proportion of recombinants over the total of recombinants and non-recombinants is identical with $\hat{\theta}$ obtained by the lod score method. Generally, however, such a count does not exploit all the information on the recombination fraction contained in the data so that it is preferable to estimate θ by maximizing $Z(\theta)$.

Usually, more than one laboratory investigates linkage between a particular pair of loci. The results of linkage analyses from different (independent) sources may be combined by simply adding the lod scores for a given θ value. An estimate of θ less than 0.5 may be interpreted in one of two ways. Either the true (but unknown) value of θ is equal to 0.5 and $\hat{\theta} < 0.5$ simply due to chance, or the true θ is indeed less than 0.5. The larger the maximum of the resulting total lod score, $Z(\hat{\theta})$, turns out to be, the more faith one has that indeed linkage exists between the two loci. $Z(\hat{\theta})$ is thus taken as the relevant statistic in the test of the null hypothesis of free recombination, $\theta = 0.5$, against the alternative hypothesis of linkage, $\theta < 0.5$. Linkage is considered significant when $Z(\hat{\theta})$ reaches or exceeds a value of 3, corresponding to odds for linkage of at least $1000:1$. Furthermore, values of θ with a lod score of $Z(\theta) < -2$ are considered very implausible and linkage is said to be excluded or ruled out at those implausible θ values.

3. TWO SIMPLE EXAMPLES

Consider two parents and a number of offspring, and assume two loci with alleles *A and *a at locus 1 and alleles *B and *b at locus 2. Let the father be doubly homozygous, *a*b/*a*b, and the mother doubly heterozygous, *A/*a, *B/*b (such a mating is called a double back-cross). Since in the mother it is not known which of the non-allelic genes

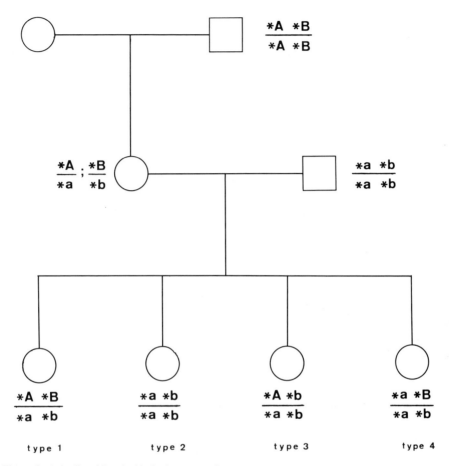

Figure 1. A family with a double back-cross mating.

are on the same chromosome (the so-called linkage phase is unknown), her genotype is either *A*B/*a*b or *A*b/*a*B. However, investigation of the phenotypes of the parents of the mother might reveal the mother's phase. If, for example, one of the mother's parents can be shown to be doubly homozygous, *A*B/*A*B or *a*b/*a*b, then this determines her genotype as *A*B/*a*b. With this genotype of the mother and that of the father given above, there are four types of offspring, *A*B/*a*b (type 1), *a*b/*a*b (type 2), *A*b/*a*b (type 3) and *a*B/*a*b (type 4). Each type has received alleles *a and *b (that is, the gamete or haplotype *a*b) from the father. Types 1 and 2 have inherited non-recombinant gametes from the mother, types 3 and 4 recombinant gametes. Let s be the number of offspring of type 1 or 2, and r be the number of offspring of type 3 or 4. Since the mother produces each of the two possible recombinant gametes with probability $\theta/2$ and each non-recombinant gamete with probability $(1-\theta)/2$, and since the offspring phenotypes occur independently of each other, s and r offspring of the given types lead to a lod score of:

$$Z(\theta) = s \log(2\theta) + r \log[2(1-\theta)]$$

23

In the example of Section 2, $r = 1$ and $s = 3$, leading to $\hat{\theta} = 0.25$ with $Z(\hat{\theta}) = 0.227$.

Assume now that the phenotypes of the grandparents and thus the linkage phase in the mother are unknown. Then, under certain regularity conditions, the two phases occur with probability of 0.5 each. Given the phase *A*B/*a*b, offspring types 1 and 2 are non-recombinants, and types 3 and 4 are recombinants, and vice versa for the phase *A*b/*a*B. The probability of occurrence of each offspring type then turns out to be equal to 1/2. However, the offspring phenotypes are no longer statistically independent (except for $\theta = 0.5$), and the lod score has to be calculated using conditional probabilities. This leads to

$$Z(\theta) = \log\{2^{r+s-1}[\theta^r(1-\theta)^s + (1-\theta)^r\theta^s]\}$$

Again assuming $r - 1$ and $s = 3$, the lod score peaks at $\hat{\theta} = 0.5$, that is such a result does not provide any evidence for linkage.

Further examples of analyses from first principles may be found in Ott (2, Section 4.1). Usually, however, it is easier to have a computer program calculate the lod scores for given values of the recombination fraction.

4. MULTI-POINT ANALYSIS

Multi-point linkage analysis refers to the simultaneous analysis of more than two gene loci, where the phenotype of each individual investigated is not necessarily known for each locus. For example, consider three loci. In addition to the recombination fraction, θ_{12}, between loci 1 and 2, one has two more recombination fractions, θ_{23} between loci 2 and 3, and θ_{13} between loci 1 and 3. One of the complications in multi-point linkage analysis consists of the potentially large number of parameters that may have to be estimated; between n gene loci, there is a total of $n(n-1)/2$ recombination fractions. Another complication refers to the order of the loci that may not be known prior to an analysis; n loci can be ordered in $n!/2 = n(n-1)(n-2)\ldots/2$ ways, when each two symmetric orders are counted as one gene order.

Experience shows that recombinations in adjacent intervals on a chromosome do not occur independently of each other. This phenomenon is called *interference* and can be observed in most living organisms. Generally, interference is negative, that is the occurrence of a recombination tends to reduce the probability for another recombination nearby. Suitable assumptions on interference allow a reduction of the number of parameters to be estimated since with a given degree of interference, recombination fractions beween adjacent loci (e.g. θ_{12}, θ_{23}) determine the recombination fractions between non-adjacent loci (e.g. θ_{13}). The proper assumptions on interference in man are still a matter of debate, but it appears that for the purpose of estimating recombination fractions, the degree of interference assumed is not crucial (and interference may thus be assumed absent) while this is much more important, for example, for the calculation of risk estimates in genetic counselling.

In general, multi-point linkage analysis by the likelihood method is a complex matter that usually requires the use of a computer program. For a given order of loci, it amounts to estimating the various recombination fractions and possibly some interference parameter by finding those parameter values associated with the largest likelihood. Repeating this procedure for different gene orders will estimate the best order, that is find that order with the largest likelihood.

Because of the complexity of multi-point likelihood analysis, several approximate methods have been described that are capable of narrowing down the large number of possible gene orders to a few plausible ones and that will possibly also find good approximations to recombination fraction estimates (8). Also, the availability of many closely linked DNA markers (RFLPs) permits efficient alternatives to the general likelihood method (9). Such alternative methods do not, however, make a general likelihood approach obsolete. For example, the only reliable and objective way to judge the plausibility of different gene orders is to compare their likelihoods. Also, generally, the calculation of genetic risks can only be carried out by computing proper likelihoods.

A particularly appealing state of affairs is the presence of several loci with known genetic distances between them, and a single locus with unknown location. In this situation, a full likelihood analysis may be carried out with a small number of parameters (10; computer program LINKMAP, Section 5). In the simplest case, the only parameter to be estimated is the distance between the locus with unknown location and one of the markers. This design represents the basis for the present search for more and more DNA markers. It is hoped that in the not too distant future, the human gene map may become so densely populated with DNA markers of known relative distances that it will be relatively easy to map any gene of unknown location, particularly disease genes (see also the Discussion in Section 10 below).

5. USING COMPUTER PROGRAMS

Quite a few computer programs exist carrying out certain tasks in linkage analysis. Some of them are designed for approximate types of linkage analyses, others pick up where a full likelihood analysis has left off, modifying or refining its results, for example, to test for heterogeneity (see 2). In this short presentation only two programs will be discussed, the LIPED program (11) and the program package called LINKAGE (10). Both calculate the likelihood of family pedigree data, given the values of various parameters such as recombination fractions, gene frequencies, etc. The LIPED program is designed for an analysis of one or two loci while the LINKAGE programs are not limited in the number of loci that may jointly be analysed. LIPED is written in Fortran, the LINKAGE programs in the Pascal language. Microcomputer versions of either program running on an IBM PC are available from me.

The LIPED program has been around for over 10 years now and has been modified to meet demands for 'user-friendliness'. Several people adapted it for special needs (for example, 12).

The LINKAGE package consists of several programs: MLINK calculates likelihoods for given parameter values, ILINK is the iterative version of MLINK and finds maximum likelihood estimates of parameters, while LINKMAP calculates likelihoods for the situation, discussed at the end of Section 4, of one locus with unknown location relative to a known map of several marker loci. The remaining two programs, PREPLINK and PEDPOINT, serve to prepare the respective locus and pedigree data such that they can be analysed by one of the three analysis programs.

To make use of these programs for an analysis of linkage, one first has to collect the relevant pedigree data. For each individual, characterized by a unique identification

(ID), one needs to know the ID of each parent, the sex of the individual and the phenotypes (possibly 'unknown') at the different loci. The phenotypes at a sex-linked locus with co-dominant alleles sometimes represent a source of confusion. For example, consider two alleles, *A and *B, and three phenotypes, *A*, *B* and *AB*, indicating whether *A is expressed, *B is expressed, or both *A and *B are expressed, respectively. Clearly, the *A* phenotype will be interpreted as the *A/*A genotype in females, and as the *A genotype in males. Users of a linkage program sometimes feel that in the input to the program, this difference has to be reflected in the representation of male and female phenotypes. However, there is no need to do this since the likelihood refers to *pheno*types, not *geno*types.

In addition to pedigree information, one also has to furnish gene frequencies and a description of the mode of inheritance at each gene locus. One possible manner to describe mode of inheritance is to define, for each genotype and each phenotype, the so-called *penetrance*, that is the conditional probability that the phenotype is expressed for a given genotype. For the example in the previous paragraph, given the *A/*A genotype, the penetrances for the three phenotypes *A*, *B* and *AB* are equal to 1, 0 and 0, respectively (in the LINKAGE programs, there is an easier way to describe such simple modes of inheritance).

While the example of the penetrances given in the previous paragraph is very simple, generally penetrances may serve as a means to tackle rather complex situations. For example, one may use them to accommodate delayed age-at-onset (see Section 6), certain kinds of epistatic associations between the phenotypes at the two loci under study (13) or genes following a Y-linked or pseudoautosomal mode of inheritance (14). In the hands of an experienced geneticist, penetrances are a powerful technical tool to adjust an analysis to very unusual situations. The following paragraph shows a particular example.

Recently, an investigator complained to me that with the available linkage programs he was lacking the possibility of using different gene frequencies for individuals with different ethnic background. Using existing programs, several solutions to this problem exist, one of them being the following. Consider a gene locus with alleles *A and *a and respective gene frequencies of 0.4 and 0.6. For a few of the individuals marrying into a pedigree (so-called originals or founders), however, the gene frequencies should be equal to 0.1 and 0.9 rather than 0.4 and 0.6. The mode of inheritance at this locus is assumed dominant, where the phenotype *A* represents expression of the *A allele, and the phenotype *NA* denotes absence of *A. The corresponding penetrances of zero and one are shown in columns one and two of *Table 1*. One may now take advantage of the fact that in the calculation of the likelihood the genotype probabilities are multiplied by the penetrances to obtain the phenotype probabilities. For the regular founder members, genotype probabilities of 0.16, 0.48 and 0.36 can be calculated from the gene frequencies of 0.4 and 0.6. For the special originals with different ethnic backgrounds, however, one should have genotype probabilities of 0.01, 0.18 and 0.81, corresponding to gene frequencies of 0.1 and 0.9. Rather than adjusting gene frequencies (which is not possible in present programs for a few exceptional individuals only), one may with the same result use the penetrances as multipliers for the genotype probabilities. For example, to transform 0.16 into 0.01, a multiplier of $1/16 = 0.0625$ is required. To implement these multipliers in a linkage program, one may for the special originals

Table 1. Penetrances used as multipliers to adjust gene frequencies for special originals with different ethnic background (see text in Section 5).

Genotype	All individuals except special originals		Special originals	
	A	NA	A	NA
*A/*A	1	0	0.0625	0
*A/*a	1	0	0.3750	0
*a/*a	0	1	0	2.25

A and *NA* denote phenotypes, *A and *a represent alleles.

(only for these individuals) replace the penetrances in the first two columns of *Table 1* by those shown in the last two columns. This has the same effect as if a different set of gene frequencies had been specified for the special originals.

When the recombination fraction, θ, is estimated by the method shown above, one assumes that recombination in male parents is the same as that in female parents, $\theta_m = \theta_f$. If one is not willing to make this assumption, the two parameters θ_m and θ_f will have to be estimated separately by finding the highest lod score in a plane of parameters with coordinate axes θ_m and θ_f. The likelihood is then no longer represented as a one-dimensional curve but rather as a mountainous surface above a plane. Parameters other than recombination fractions may also be estimated using linkage programs but this will not be pursued any further here.

The execution time of a linkage program depends very much on the problem to be analysed. Everything else being equal, running time is approximately proportional to the number of genotypes, considered jointly at all loci. This is, however, only a very rough approximation that holds only when the phenotypes do not exhibit the genotypes well. Under these assumptions, consider the following examples. When m and n are the number of alleles at locus 1 and 2, respectively then the number of joint genotypes is equal to $mn(mn + 1)/2$. It is easy to verify that for $m > 1$ and $n > 1$, doubling the number of alleles at locus 1 will lead to an increase in the number of genotypes by a factor of between 3.6 and 4. It can be expected that execution time will also be increased by about this factor. Similarly, under comparable conditions, a three-point analysis with three alleles at each locus will take about as much time to run as a two-point analysis with nine and three alleles. In efficiently designed programs, increasing the number of alleles or loci will not generally lead to such a drastic increase in execution time.

6. REDUCED PENETRANCE

In simple modes of inheritance, the penetrances (see Section 5) take on values of zero or one. For example, consider two alleles, *A and *a, and two phenotypes, *A* (*A is expressed) and *NA* (not *A*). For the genotype *A/*A, let the penetrances be 1 and 0, and for the genotype *a/*a, assume penetrances of 0 and 1 (the order $A - NA$ is assumed for the phenotypes). Depending on the penetrances for the heterozygous genotype, *A/*a, the mode of inheritance is dominant or recessive. If these are equal to 1 and 0, then *A is dominant over the *a allele, and for penetrances of 0 and 1 (corresponding to the phenotypes *A* and *NA*), then *A is recessive with respect to *a.

In many situations, however, it is unrealistic to assume penetrances of 0 and 1. For example, one may sometimes misclassify an unaffected individual as affected and vice versa. Then, such a classification error may, for example, be reflected by penetrances of 0.05 and 0.95 rather than of 0 and 1.

A well-known case of reduced penetrance is age-dependent penetrances, or delayed age at onset of a disease. Several diseases caused by a single gene are not expressed at birth but are manifested only later in life. Then each age category may be character-ized by its own set of penetrances. If the disease penetrance for a susceptible individual (i.e. one carrying the disease gene) is close to zero at birth, it may rise gradually to attain a value of close to one at greater age. Often, such an age-at-onset curve shows a sigmoid shape. For the purpose of estimating the recombination fraction, it appears that the exact shape of the curve is not very relevant and that even a sloped straight line, although clearly inaccurate, will usually yield accurate estimates of the recombi-nation. However, it has to be pointed out that a correct determination of age-dependent penetrances is important, for example, in the calculation of genetic risks.

7. POINT AND INTERVAL ESTIMATES

The recombination estimates obtained by the lod score method are so-called maximum likelihood (ML) estimates. These can be shown to have the following properties (for a detailed discussion, see 2). Except in simple situations such as those allowing for a count of recombinants and non-recombinants, recombination fraction estimates are *biased*, that is the weighted average of all estimates possibly occurring differs from the true value of the recombination fraction. In some cases, the bias can be quite pro-nounced, particularly with small numbers of observations. Generally, however, the bias of ML estimates becomes smaller with increasing sample size; bias as well as variance of the estimates tends to vanish for a sample size tending to infinity, that is ML estimates are generally *consistent*. Furthermore, with a large number of obser-vations, ML estimates are approximately normally distributed with a variance that can be estimated from the curvature of the likelihood or lod score and thus allows the calcu-lation of approximate confidence intervals.

In addition to point estimates of recombination fractions and other parameters, it is useful to obtain some idea of the variability or reliability of these estimates, that is one would like to also compute interval estimates. To this end, several methods are available. One method exploits the approximate normality of ML estimates to obtain approximate confidence intervals or, for more than one parameter estimated jointly, approximate confidence regions bounded by ellipses or ellipsoids. Practical calcula-tions are given in (2).

Another method to judge the reliability of ML estimates is to construct so-called sup-port intervals, where support denotes the logarithm of the likelihood. As the term 'sup-port' is not in general use among geneticists, such intervals are usually also called approximate confidence intervals. As recommended by the Committee on Methods of Linkage Analysis and Reporting, Eighth Human Gene Mapping Workshop (7), for a single estimate of the recombination fraction, approximate confidence intervals are con-structed as follows. Consider a ML estimate, $\hat{\theta}$, from which the curve of the lod score, $Z(\theta)$, falls off. Imagine a horizontal straight line drawn at a vertical distance of one unit of lod score below the maximum lod, $Z(\hat{\theta})$. The points of intersection between this horizontal line and the lod score curve define the end points of the approximate confidence interval for θ that, roughly speaking, has an associated confidence coefficient of 95% and, in small samples, of at least 90%.

In addition to recommending the above type of confidence interval for a single recombination fraction, the same committee has strongly advocated the calculation of separate lod score for males and females. This is usually done by reporting the 'marginal' lod scores, $Z(\theta_m, \theta_f = 0.5)$ and $Z(\theta_m = 0.5, \theta_f)$, that is the lod scores for one sex when the recombination fraction for the other sex is kept at 0.5. Some caution is required in the use of this method and more satisfactory but more complicated methods are discussed in reference (2).

Based on parameter estimates obtained by the likelihood method, one often calculates derived quantities that are functions of these parameters. For example, an analysis may show heterogeneity suggesting the presence of two types of families, one type with linkage between the two loci analysed, and another type without linkage. In this situation, one will estimate two parameters, the proportion, α, of families of the linked type, and the recombination fraction, θ, in these families. The posterior probability, w_i, that the i-th family belongs to the linked type, is then a function of both α and θ. An approximate confidence interval for w_i may be obtained by the simple principle (reference 2, p. 193) that whenever a pair of values (α, θ) is inside its confidence region, then the value of w_i computed from (α, θ) is taken to belong to the confidence interval for the posterior probability of linkage for the i-th family. An application of this method to some families with Huntington's disease is given in Ott (15).

8. HETEROGENEITY WITH TWO-POINT AND MULTI-POINT DATA

In linkage analysis, disease heterogeneity is manifested by a difference in the recombination fraction between disease and marker loci in different families. A plausible explanation for this would usually be that the same disease phenotype is caused by different mechanisms in different families. Consider two-point situations first. Under homogeneity, the recombination fraction, θ, between disease locus and genetic marker is the same in each family although, of course, the estimates, $\hat{\theta}$, may fluctuate between families. Two kinds of alternatives to homogeneity have been considered. In the test for heterogeneity by Morton (16), the recombination fraction is potentially different in each family. On the other hand, in the A-test, two types of families are assumed, one type with linkage and one type without linkage, where α is the proportion of linked families and θ is the recombination fraction in the linked families (see last paragraph of Section 7). Both tests are easy to carry out (2); for the A-test, a small computer program, HOMOG, is available from me.

With more than two loci, consider the situation of a known map of marker loci (this may be an approximation to reality) and of a disease locus about whose location conflicting results have been reported. The question arises whether one faces a case of heterogeneity, that is whether two (or more) diseases exist that happen to show the same clinical picture and that are caused by genes at different locations on the gene map. A multi-point test for heterogeneity may be carried out as follows. Let x be the genetic distance between the disease locus and a fixed locus of the marker loci. The likelihood, $L(x)$, for the relative location of the disease locus with respect to the map of the marker loci may conveniently be calculated by the LINKMAP program (Section 4, last paragraph). Different family pedigrees may now yield different estimates of genetic distance; some may even place the disease locus in different map intervals than others. Under heterogeneity, the maximum log likelihood is given by the sum, S_1, of the log $L(\hat{x}_i)$, where $\hat{x}_i$ is the ML estimate of the genetic distance in the i-th family. Under homogeneity, the maximum log likelihood, S_0, is equal to log $L(\hat{x})$, that is the maximum of the sum over all *n* families of the log likelihood. Ordinarily, $2(S_1 - S_0)$ is taken to approximately follow a chi-square distribution on $n-1$ degrees of freedom and is used to test the hypothesis of homogeneity. This procedure may, however, not be reliable when different gene orders are involved. Alternatively, one may declare a difference $S_1 - S_0$ as relevant when it exceeds a value of 2, say. Along similar lines, a multi-point test of homogeneity may be constructed for the alternative of only two types of families, each type being characterized by a fixed value of genetic distance to be estimated.

9. GENETIC RISKS

In some mongenic diseases, susceptible individuals (i.e. those carrying the disease gene) express the trait only later in life. An individual at risk, that is an individual who potentially has inherited the disease gene, may want to know the chance that he or she has in fact inherited the disease gene. Such genetic risks can be calculated as conditional probabilities , given all the phenotypic information on the individual and the relatives.

A very simple example is the following. Consider a marker locus with alleles *A and *B, linked with recombination fraction, θ, to a disease locus. Assume that one parent carries the disease gene, is doubly heterozygous for the marker locus, and that the phase is known such that in this parent the disease gene is on the same chromosome as the *A allele and the normal gene is on the same chromosome as the *B allele. Then, for an offspring who inherited the *A allele, the probability also to have inherited the disease allele is equal to $1 - \theta$. The point and interval estimates (Section 7) of the genetic risk are then easily obtained from the estimates of θ.

Usually, however, the genetic risk is a rather complicated function of θ and of other parameters such as gene frequencies. In three-point linkage, when the disease locus may be flanked by two marker loci, the risk is generally a complicated function of the two recombination fractions, θ_{12} and θ_{23}. Point and interval estimates of the risk may then be obtained by the methods discussed in Section 7.

The practical calculation of a risk figure is generally quite difficult. Although for simple family types one may apply formalized rules working with prior, conditional and posterior probabilities, it appears safer to proceed with conventional probability calculus where feasible. An elegant approach to calculating genetic risks is due to Elston and Stewart (6). Assume that one needs to calculate the conditional probability, given all pedigree data, that an individual in the pedigree (possibly an unborn child) has genotype *g*. Then, this probability is simply given by $L(g)/L$, where L is the pedigree likelihood (possibly obtained from a computer program) and $L(g)$ is the likelihood under the assumption that the individual has genotype *g*. This approach is usually easy to apply, but some care is required in the calculation of $L(g)$, particularly in the presence of reduced or age-dependent penetrance. Then, as mentioned in Section 6, proper penetrance values are important for genetic risks while this is much less the case for the estimation of the recombination fraction.

The MLINK computer program in the LINKAGE program package (10) has a built-in option for the calculation of genetic risks. The method applied is based on the ability of the program to 'peel' (recursively calculate) the likelihood onto any individual in the pedigree. This feature virtually eliminates any computational problems in the derivation of genetic risks.

10. DISCUSSION

Likelihood analyses of genetic linkage as usually carried out involve the following two tacit assumptions that have not been discussed so far.

(i) The only source of variation allowed in the phenotypes is due to single genes and random environmental influences. In particular, absence of polygenic background is assumed. While this does not represent any problem for many genetic markers such as RFLPs, it might do so for diseases. However, the success of present linkage analysis suggests that this restriction is not too serious.

(ii) For loci to be analysed for linkage, absence of epistatic interaction between the phenotypes at different loci is assumed. For certain types of epistatic interactions, methods have been developed so that one can get around this restriction (13). However, tight linkage with gamete disequilibrium can be shown to be indistinguishable from epistasis even in large pedigrees (17). Therefore, depending on the linkage problem, the assumption of no epistatic interaction can be felt to represent a serious restriction.

While linkage analysis has been very successful as one of the tools of gene mapping, for very short genetic distances it does not appear to be the method of choice. The reason for this is 2-fold. For one thing, with very small distances, a rather large number of observations (opportunities for recombination) is required for an appreciable chance to observe a recombination. More seriously, recent discoveries of recombination hot spots might suggest that recombination predominantly occurs at a limited number of points on the genome, with a much reduced frequency between these points, which renders linkage analysis too crude a tool for fine-mapping (18).

Two major objectives of linkage analysis are (i) mapping the human genome and (ii) providing improved risk estimates in genetic counselling. While the various methods of molecular biology and somatic cell genetics furnish physical distances between points on the human gene map, linkage analysis yields genetic distances. These are also the relevant quantities in genetic counselling.

11. REFERENCES

1. Conneally,P.M. and Rivas,M.L. (1980) In *Advances in Human Genetics,* Vol. **10**, Harris,H. and Hirschhorn,K. (eds.), Plenum, New York, p. 209.
2. Ott,J. (1985) *Analysis of Human Genetic Linkage,* Johns Hopkins University Press, Baltimore.
3. Botstein,D., White,R.L., Skolnick,M. and Davis,R.W. (1980) *Am. J. Hum. Genet.,* **32**, 314.
4. Haldane,J.B.S. and Smith,C.A.B. (1947) *Ann. Eugenet.,* **14**, 10.
5. Morton,N.E. (1955) *Am. J. Hum. Genet.,* **7**, 277.
6. Elston,R.C. and Stewart,J. (1971) *Hum. Hered.,* **21**, 523.
7. Conneally,P.M., Edwards,J.H., Kidd,K.K., Lalouel,J.M., Morton,N.E., Ott,J. and White,R. (1985) *Cytogenet. Cell Genet.,* **40**, 356.

8. MacCluer,J.W., Falk,C.T. and Wagener,D.K. (1985) *Genet. Epidemiol.*, in press.
9. Thompson,E.A. (1986) *Genet. Epidemiol.*, in press.
10. Lathrop,G.M., Lalouel,J.M., Julier,C. and Ott,J. (1984) *Proc. Natl. Acad. Sci. USA.*, **81**, 3443.
11. Ott,J. (1974) *Am. J. Hum. Genet.*, **26**, 588.
12. Hodge,S.E., Morton,L.A., Tideman,S., Kidd,K.K. and Spence,M.A. (1979) *Am. J. Hum. Genet.*, **31**, 761.
13. Ott,J. and Falk,C.T. (1982) *Hum. Genet.*, **62**, 296.
14. Ott,J. (1986) *Am. J. Hum. Genet.*, in press.
15. Ott,J. (1986) *Genet. Epidemiol.*, in press.
16. Morton,N.E. (1956) *Am. J. Hum. Genet.*, **8**, 80.
17. Clerget-Darpoux,F. and Lathrop,G.M. (1985) *Hum. Genet.*, **69**, 188.
18. Bodmer,W.F. (1984) In *Histocompatibility Testing 1984*, Albert,E.D., Baur,M.P. and Mayr,W.R. (eds.), Springer, Berlin-Heidelberg, p. 11.

CHAPTER 3

The use of synthetic oligonucleotides as specific hybridization probes in the diagnosis of genetic disorders

SWEE LAY THEIN and R. BRUCE WALLACE

1. INTRODUCTION

Within the last few years the method of restriction enzyme analysis, Southern blotting and mixed phase hybridization has become a technique fundamental to the analysis of human genetic disorders. It has certainly proved indispensable for carrier detection and prenatal diagnosis by DNA analysis. However, there is one severe limitation of this technique and that is it cannot directly detect the majority of mutations as these are point mutations which do not involve restriction enzyme cleavage sites. These point mutations can only be identified indirectly by linkage analysis to polymorphic restriction enzyme sites near the gene (1).

For practical purposes, point mutations can be considered to be single base substitutions or minor insertions or deletions. To detect these changes in the DNA sequence of the whole genome directly on the basis of hybridization, the size of the DNA probe used is critical. It has to be short enough to differentiate between a perfectly matched hybrid and one with a single base mismatch and yet long enough so that the sequence detected is unique in the whole genome. The DNA probes used in the routine Southern blotting analysis are generally so long that their hybridization is insensitive to minor differences between probe and template.

In a study of the effect of single base pair mismatches on the hybridization behaviour of oligonucleotides, Wallace and co-workers observed that the duplexes with a single base pair mismatch which were formed when 11, 14 or 17 base long oligonucleotides were hybridized to ϕX174 DNA were significantly less stable (dissociated at a lower temperature) than their perfectly matched counterparts (2). This difference in thermal stability made it possible by the appropriate choice of hybridization temperature to eliminate the formation of mismatched duplexes without affecting the formation of perfectly matched ones. Since mutation in a single base would affect the hybridization behaviour of an oligonucleotide complementary to the DNA sequence in the region of the mutation, oligonucleotide hybridization has the potential to provide a method for detecting single base changes within genomic DNA. The oligonucleotide has to be long enough so that the sequence detected has a probability of occurring only once in the genome; this minimum length has been calculated to be 17 nucleotides for the human genome (3).

The methodology of oligonucleotide hybridization has been developed and successfully used in the diagnosis of single base changes in sickle cell disease (4), various β-thalassaemias (5−7), α_1-anti-trypsin deficiency (8) and, more recently, point mutations in malignancies (9). However, this represents only one of the numerous applications of synthetic oligonucleotides; the use of synthetic DNA primers in DNA sequencing, as probes in the isolation of genes and in site-direct mutagenesis, has long been established (10−13). This chapter does not attempt to cover all the various applications but concentrates on the practical aspects of synthetic oligonucleotides as specific hybridization probes for the detection of point mutations in human genomic DNA. The method outlined below is currently employed in our laboratories and, whenever possible, alternatives have been included.

2. PRINCIPLES OF OLIGONUCLEOTIDE HYBRIDIZATION

2.1 **Hybridization parameters**

The use of synthetic oligonucleotides as hybridization probes is based on two principles.

(i)   That these molecules are capable of forming hydrogen bonds with complementary DNA or RNA sequences giving rise to their extremely specific hybridization behaviour.

(ii)   That the oligonucleotide−complementary DNA duplex formation is reversible.

2.1.1 *Hybrid stability*

The stability of a DNA duplex formation depends on several factors including temperature, ionic strength, base composition, the length of the duplex, the presence of any destabilizing agents and the presence of any mismatched base pairs (14). [Mismatched base pairs refer to any case where the base in one of the DNA strands cannot form a Watson/Crick base pair with the base in the complementary strand.] An index of this stability is given by the melting temperature (Tm, temperature at which 50% of the duplexes are dissociated) which is a function of the various factors mentioned. The higher the Tm the more stable the duplex. In the case of oligonucleotide probes, by comparing the dissociation of several oligonucleotide−DNA complexes as a function of temperature, an empirical formula has been derived (15) for the dissociation temperature (Td), the temperature at which half of the duplexes are dissociated.

$$T\text{d (°C)} = 4 \text{ (G +C)} + 2(\text{A + T})$$

where G, C, A and T indicate the number of the corresponding nucleotides in the oligomer. This relationship is valid only for perfectly matched duplexes beween 11 and 20 bases long in 1 M Na$^+$ and serves as a guide for determining an appropriate hybridization temperature. For hybrids shorter than 20 bp the Td decreases between 5 and 10°C for every mismatched base pair. Thus, a temperature 5°C below the Td is generally used to select for the formation of perfectly matched duplexes, those with one or more mismatched base pairs do not form (16).

Therefore, in oligonucleotide probe hybridization, the stringency is altered by adjusting the temperature, the ionic strength being kept constant at 1 M Na$^+$. The stringency can be adjusted either during hybridization or in the post-hybridization washes. To determine the appropriate temperature, it is often convenient to perform hybridization at reduced stringency and wash at increasing stringencies, analysing the results after each wash. In the initial stages of working out the conditions for the oligonucleotide probes, the optimum temperature would have been determined using cloned DNA controls. In such cases, hybridization reactions should be performed under the most stringent conditions possible in order to minimize hybridization of the probe to related but non-identical sequences.

Recently, a technique which uses tetramethylammonium chloride (Me$_4$NCl) to eliminate the dependence of Td on the G.C content of the probe was described (17). Me$_4$NCl binds selectively to A.T base pairs eliminating the preferential melting of A.T versus G.C base pairs, allowing the stringency of the hybridization to be controlled as a function of probe length only. In this procedure, an initial non-stringent hybridization with the radiolabelled oligonucleotide is followed by washing twice for 20 min each with 3.0 M Me$_4$NCl to control the stringency of the hybridization. Although the method may be advantageous for screening a complex library with a pool of oligonucleotide probes, it offers little advantage when a pair of oligonucleotides with a known Td is used.

2.1.2 *Hybridization kinetics*

The time required for duplex formation with an immobilized target sequence is much shorter for synthetic oligonucleotide probes than that for complementary probes (e.g. those generated by nick translations). This is due to the fact that much higher molar concentrations of probe are available in the case of oligonucleotide probes. Unlike complementary probes where probe reannealing in solution can decrease the concentration of probe available for hybridization with the target, synthetic oligonucleotide hybridization probes are single-stranded and available in vast excess over that of the target sequences. The rate of hybridization of oligonucleotide probe to DNA immobilized on a solid matrix follows first-order kinetics with respect to oligonucleotide concentration. The time ($t_{1/2}$) required for half the probe to anneal with the immobilized DNA sequences is:

$$t_{1/2} = \frac{\ln 2}{kC} \qquad \text{(see ref. 18)}$$

Where k = first-order rate constant (litres mol nucleotide^{-1} sec^{-1})

C = probe concentration (mol nucleotide/litre)

The rate constant (k) as a function of length and complexity of the probes has been described by Wetmur and Davidson (19) as

$$k = 3.5 \times 10^5 \times L^{0.5} \times N^{-1} \text{ mol nucleotide}^{-1} \text{ sec}^{-1}$$

Where L = length of the probe in nucleotides

N = complexity of the probe; i.e. number of nucleotides in non-repeating sequence for hybridizations done in 1 M Na$^+$ and is applicable to oligonucleotides as short as 11 bp (2). Therefore, the time (in seconds) required to anneal half of the probe to the target sequence is given by:

$$t_{1/2} = \frac{N \ln 2}{3.5 \times 10^5 \times L^{0.5} \times C}$$

The hybridization time for synthetic oligonucleotide probes is minimized as they are of low complexity and present in vast excess. Thus, for a probe with a complexity (and length) of 15 bp present at 10 ng/ml (3×10^{-8} mol nucleotides/litre), the hybridization is half complete ($t_{1/2}$) in 250 sec and 99.6% complete in 33 min.

Another difference in the hybridization behaviour of oligonucleotide probes from that of nick-translated probes is the effect of dextran sulphate on the hybridization rate. The rate of hybridization is increased up to 100-fold for hybridization using nick-translated probes in dextran sulphate (20) whereas dextran sulphate has a minimal effect on the hybridization rate of short oligonucleotides. This difference is attributed to the ability of the molecules generated by nick-translation to form probe 'networks' between their partially overlapping sequences. The short oligonucleotides are single-stranded and thus do not form such networks.

2.2 Oligonucleotide probe design

In their application as specific hybridization probes for the detection of point mutations, synthetic oligonucleotides are used in pairs; one oligonucleotide is completely homologous to the normal gene sequence, the other to the mutant gene sequence at a region around the point mutation. The two probes differ from each other by a single nucleotide (in the case where they are complementary to the same DNA strand). When these oligonucleotides are synthesized, three aspects of the DNA sequence must be considered. These include

(i)   oligonucleotide length;
(ii)   G (guanines) + C (cytosines) content;
(iii)   the presence of non-complementary bases.

2.2.1 *Length*

Basically, the length of the oligonucleotide probe determines its hybridization specificity. The longer a sequence, the more likely it is to be unique amongst the collection of sequences the oligonucleotide is used to probe. The length is limited more by need than by synthetic considerations since deoxyoligonucleotides up to 100 bases long can now be prepared rapidly and in high yield with the recent advances in nucleic acid chemistry.

To be unique the oligonucleotide probe must contain at least 'N' nucleotides where

$$4^N > 2 \times \text{no. of base pairs in the target genome} \qquad \text{(see ref. 3)}$$

The haploid human genome contains 3×10^9 bases, giving N a value of 17. Therefore, an oligonucleotide has to be at least 17 bases long before it can be used as a specific hybridization probe for the human genome.

Another method of determining the minimum length of the oligoprobe required is to calculate the expected frequency (a) of length l:

$$a = \frac{g}{2} l_1 \times \frac{1-g}{2} l_2 \qquad \text{(see ref. 21)}$$

Where   g   = fractional G + C content of the human genome
l_1 = number of G + C in the sequence (l) to be probed
l_2 = number of (A) adenines plus (T) thymines
         in sequence l ($1 = l_2 + l_2$)

To detect a 19-base long sequence with an eight G + C content in the sequence, the expected number of oligonucleotide-complementary sites (n) is:

$$n = 2 \times \text{size of haploid genome} \times a$$
$$n = 2 \times 3 \times 10^9 \times a$$
$$= 2 \times 10^{-2}$$

In addition to specificity, oligonucleotide length determines duplex stability (2). Sequences shorter than 11 bases have been found to give unacceptable results as probes for cloned DNAs (16). In deciding the length of the oligonucleotide probe, one has to take into consideration the effect of mismatches on the duplex stability to obtain the optimum difference in hybridization between mismatched duplexes and perfectly matched ones. Previous experience has shown that the optimum length of oligonucleotide for detection of a single base mismatch is 19 bases.

2.2.2 *G + C content*

It has long been established that the higher the GC content of a duplex the greater the duplex stability. Although no detailed thermodynamic study has been done, an empirical relationship of the G + C content on duplex stability (given by the parameter Td) has been derived for oligonucleotides $11-20$ bases long in 1 M Na^+.

$$Td = 4(G + C) + 2(A + T)$$

This relationship is useful for estimating the effects of length and G + C content on duplex stability (for detailed analysis, see review by Smith, 11), as well as for determining an appropriate hybridization temperature (15) (see earlier discussion).

In addition to effects on the duplex stability, the G content of oligonucleotides has an effect on the DNA synthesis itself, particularly on purification of the oligonucleotide. G-rich oligonucleotides are notoriously difficult to purify. Although purification schemes have been devised (22), it is best to avoid the problem if possible. This is often achieved by simply synthesizing the complementary sequence. This would often serve the same purpose for many applications. Alternatively, an oligonucleotide complementary to a different region is synthesized.

2.2.3 *Presence of non-complementary bases*

The presence of a single base pair mismatch will reduce the stability of oligonucleotide − DNA duplexes and this effect depends on two factors:

(i)   Position of the mismatch relative to the end of the duplex. Studies have shown that the duplex with a central mismatch is least stable. To achieve the destabilizing effect the mismatch should be at least five nucleotides from either end of a 19 base long oligonucleotide − DNA duplex.

(ii)   Type of mismatch.

Wallace and co-workers have studied the effects of the different types of mismatched base pairs (A−C, T−T, A−A, G−T) on the stability of oligonucleotide−DNA duplexes (2,15,23). Although the destabilization effects have not been quantitatively demonstrated, the relative stability of G−T versus A−C mismatches has been observed in several applications. Therefore, to obtain the maximum destabilizing effect, a G−T mismatch should be avoided whenever possible, and this is achieved by simply synthesizing the complementary sequence producing an A−C mismatch instead. Similarly, it has recently been found that A−G mismatches are more stable than T−C mismatches and thus A−G should be avoided where possible (Wallace and Schold, unpublished).

For hybridization conditions under which duplexes with one or more mismatches will not form, Suggs *et al.* (15) have suggested a hybridization temperature of 2−5°C below the calculated T_d in 1 M Na$^+$. However, conditions for eliminating mismatch hybridizations must be determined empirically for each oligonucleotide. Problems may be encountered with GC-rich oligonucleotide duplexes due to their enhanced stability.

It has also been shown that single mismatched duplexes can form at lower temperatures and that such hybridization occurs at specific complementary sites (2). Since the rate of formation of single base pair mismatched duplexes is the same as perfectly matched ones, it remains that the rate of dissociation of these duplexes must differ to account for the differential hybridization behaviour. The consequence of this differential dissociation rate is that the time used in the post-hybridization wash is very critical. This is further discussed in the technical section.

3. DETECTION OF TARGET DNA SEQUENCE

A summary of the procedure is outlined in *Figure 1*. Genomic DNA is digested with an appropriate restriction enzyme. The DNA fragments are then separated according

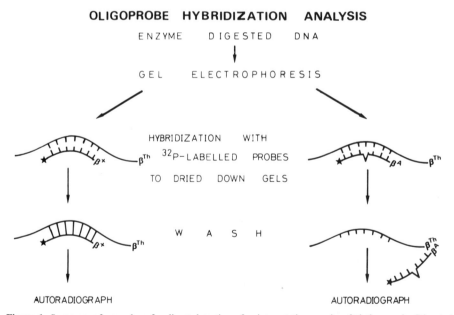

Figure 1. Summary of procedure for direct detection of point mutation causing β-thalassaemia. Digested genomic DNA is fractionated on agarose gel electrophoresis, then denatured and immobilized '*in situ*' by drying down the agarose gel. Oligonucleotide probe (β$^+$) which corresponds to the β-thalassaemic sequence forms a perfect hybrid with the β-thalassaemic gene while the normal oligonucleotide probe (β^A) forms a single base mismatched hybrid with the β-thalassaemic gene. Under the appropriate hybridization and washing conditions the mismatched hybrid dissociates while the perfectly matched hybrid remains and can be detected by autoradiography.

to size on agarose gel electrophoresis and immobilized either '*in situ*' by drying down the gel or transferred by Southern blotting onto a membrane. A duplicate gel is run in parallel; one gel is hybridized to the oligonucleotide probe with the normal sequence and the other to the probe with the mutant sequence. Under the appropriate hybridization and washing conditions the hybrid with a single base mismatch dissociates while the perfectly matched hybrid remains and can be detected by autoradiography.

3.1 Choosing the right restriction enzyme

In oligonucleotide hybridization of genomic DNA, high molecular weight non-specific hybridization is usually observed; the extent depending on the length and complexity of the oligonucleotide probe and the restriction enzyme digest. DNA digested with an enzyme which cuts frequently has less high molecular weight fragments and reduced smearing from the non-specific hybridization. Genomic DNA is digested with an appropriate restriction enzyme chosen such that the unique sequence to be probed is present within a restriction fragment of 1.5−3.5 kb in size, clearly discernible from the high molecular weight DNA smearing. The latter can also be reduced by digesting the genomic DNA with a second enzyme which cuts outside the desired fragment, thereby increasing fragmentation of the genomic DNA, but leaving the desired fragment intact.

Occasionally low molecular weight cross-hybridizing bands are seen (7). Their origin is not clear; they vary with different oligonucleotide probes but for each oligonucleotide the position is constant. They do not interfere with the interpretation of the results and are extremely useful as internal controls for the quantitation and assessment of completeness of digestion of DNA.

3.2 Immobilization of DNA — dried agarose gel versus membrane

The DNA fragments generated by the appropriate restriction endonuclease are separated according to size by agarose gel electrophoresis, denatured '*in situ*' and then can be immobilized in the agarose gel itself by drying down or onto a membrane by Southern blot transfer (24). Dried agarose gel is used as a personal preference for the following reasons.

(i)   Oligonucleotide probes hybridize about 5-fold more effectively with DNA fragments in agarose gels than with fragments transferred to nitrocellulose (N/C) (25). This is probably due to decreased hybrid stability caused by some bases which are prevented from forming hydrogen bonds because they are bound to or sterically hindered by the solid support. The efficiency of detecting DNA fragments is also improved because transfer of DNA fragments is not involved.

(ii) Unlike N/C or other membranes, dried agarose gels can be repeatedly subjected to post-hybridization washes following the initial wash and exposure until the optimum signal-to-background noise ratio is obtained. N/C, however, once dried after the post-hybridization, often retains any background non-specific radioactivity. This difference is probably because oligonucleotides can easily diffuse into and out of the gel matrix.

(iii) Time of the procedure is reduced because no transfer of DNA fragments is involved and pre-hybridization of agarose gels has been found to be unnecessary.

However, it is still necessary to pre-hybridize N/C to reduce the non-specific background hybridization.

(iv)   A possible disadvantage of agarose gels is the loss of the smaller DNA fragments but with the short hybridization times required for oligonucleotide probes this loss is minimized.

(v)   Dried agarose gels could also be repeatedly re-hybridized with different probes after elution of the previous probe by alkali treatment.

3.3 Oligonucleotide probe preparation

The oligonucleotides are radiolabelled before they can be used as probes. The method used depends mainly on the sensitivity required.

3.3.1 *Radiolabelling of oligonucleotides*

Oligonucleotides synthesized by the phosphotriester approach can be purified as either the 5' OH- or 5' dimethoxytrityl (DMT)-containing molecule. There are two methods of radiolabelling the oligonucleotides.

(i) *5' ^{32}P-end labelling.* This method suffices for most applications of oligoprobe hybridization. It involves the transfer of ^{32}P from [γ-^{32}P]ATP to the 5' end of the oligonucleotide in exchange for the OH (hydroxyl) group using T4 polynucleotide kinase (26). As only one molecule of ^{32}P is incorporated into one molecule of oligonucleotide, the maximum specific activity of the oligoprobe attainable would be that of the [γ-^{32}P]ATP used.

(ii) *3' Primer extension.* This method as described by Studencki and Wallace (25) produces oligonucleotide probes of extremely high specific activity. In this method two oligonucleotides are used in one of two strategies (*Figure 2*). In scheme I, one oligonucleotide which serves as a template is combined with a shorter primer which is complementary to the 3' end of the template. In scheme II, both oligonucleotides serve as primer and template. In either case, the primer/template complex is extended with DNA polymerase I (Klenow fragment) in the presence of [α-^{32}P]dNTPs (deoxynucleoside triphosphates). For subsequent strand separation, it is convenient if the primer contains a 5' DMT and the template a 5' phosphate. The specific activity of the oligonucleotide probe produced varies with the number of [α-^{32}P]dNTPs incorporated; [α-^{32}P]dATP has been used with dCTP, dGTP and dTTP in the labelling of oligomers for the detection of mutations of the N-*ras* gene (27). The extremely high specific activities of oligonucleotide probes produced when all four [α-^{32}P]dNTPs are used (5 − 10 times those achieved by the kinase reaction), makes it possible to detect single-copy gene sequences in as little as 1 μg of genomic DNA (25). In addition, the approach has several unique advantages. First, using scheme II a longer oligonucleotide probe can be generated from two shorter ones. Secondly, modified nucleosides (e.g. biotinylated deoxyuridine, 28) can be incorporated into the duplex if desired. Thirdly, isotopes other than ^{32}P can be incorporated (e.g. ^{35}S, ^{125}I, ^{3}H, etc.).

3.3.2 *Separation of radiolabelled probe*

The sensitivity of detection of a certain DNA sequence is dependent on the specific

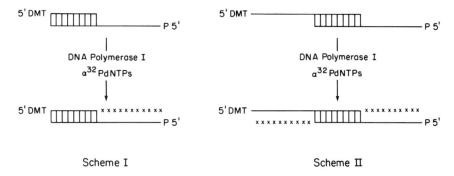

Scheme I   Scheme II

Figure 2. Labelling by 3′ primer extenstion. **Scheme I:** an oligonucleotide template and primer (seven bases or longer) are combined in equal molar amounts and extended with DNA polymerase I (Klenow fragment) in the presence of $[\alpha\text{-}^{32}\text{P}]$dNTPs (or other labelled deoxynucleoside triphosphates). If the template has a 5′ phosphate and the extended product a 5′ OH or 5′ DMT, they can be strand separated by thin layer chromatography or polyacrylamide gel electrophoresis. **Scheme II:** two oligonucleotides complementary at their 3′ ends (over seven bases or longer) are combined in equal molar amounts and extended in a DNA polymerase I reaction as described in **Scheme I**.

activity that can be achieved in the radiolabelling of the probe which in turn depends on the specific activity of the $[^{32}\text{P}]$ATP used and the number of ^{32}P atoms that can be incorporated into the probe. Thus the specific activity of 5′ end-labelled oligonucleotide probes is severely limited by the specific activity of the $[\gamma\text{-}^{32}\text{P}]$ATP itself, because only one ^{32}P atom can be incorporated. It is therefore extremely important not only to separate the labelled ('hot') oligonucleotides from the unincorporated $[\gamma\text{-}^{32}\text{P}]$ATP but also to ensure that probe hybridization to the target genomic sequences is not reduced by any contaminating unlabelled ('cold') oligonucleotide. A clean separation of the labelled oligonucleotide from the unincorporated $[\gamma\text{-}^{32}\text{P}]$ATP or $[\alpha\text{-}^{32}\text{P}]$dNTPs and the unlabelled oligonucleotide can be achieved by (i) thin layer chromatography or (ii) polyacrylamide gel electrophoresis in the presence of 7 M urea. The latter method is routinely used in our laboratories and is described in detail below; in this method the separation depends on the different mobilities of the 5′ phosphorylated oligonucleotide, the 5′ OH oligonucleotide and the 5′DMT oligonucleotide (25).

Other methods of separation of the labelled strand which have been described include chromatography on the anion exchange resin DE52 and the Bio-gel P_4 column. Both these methods give no separation of the 'hot' from the 'cold' oligonucleotide.

3.4 Hybridization conditions

3.4.1 *Pre-hybridization*

Pre-hybridization of filters containing immobilized DNA with subtances which bind to non-specific nucleic acid binding sites on the filters is prescribed as an effective means of reducing background hybridization. With oligonucleotide probes we have found it to be unnecesary in direct-gel hybridizations. However, pre-hybridization of N/C membranes does appear to have a beneficial effect. When needed, pre-hybridization can be done in a buffer containing non-specific nucleic acid sequences such as *Escherichia coli* or calf thymus DNA, yeast tRNA or oligoribonucleotides.

3.4.2 *Hybridization and washing*

All hybridization and washing manipulations of oligonucleotide probes are performed in 1 M Na^+ conditions so that the stringency is altered by the temperature and the time of post-hybridization wash. The hybridization is generally done at 5°C below the calculated Td but not higher than 70°C, for a minimum of 2 h.

Hybridization is followed by initial washes in 6 × standard saline citrate (SSC) at room temperature to remove unhybridized probes. The gel is then given a stringent wash for 1−2 min usually at 5°C below the calculated Td. This is then followed by a long wash (1−2 h) at room temperature to remove the probes that have melted from the single base mismatched duplexes.

The hybridization and washing conditions for each set of oligonucleotide probes should have been initially worked out using known DNA controls. In addition, the 'cleanliness' of the wash should be monitored with a Geiger counter. It should be realized that there will be some background hybridization with oligonucleotide probes. The important parameter is signal-to-noise ratio. Negative and, where possible, positive hybridization controls should be included in each gel. After the initial wash and exposure, additional washes can be done to reduce the background or to improve the selectivity of hybridization (e.g. to remove mismatched duplexes).

Table 1. Preparation of gel.

1.	Digest 10 µg of genomic DNA with the appropriate restriction enzyme.
2.	Electrophorese the digested DNA with an equivalent amount[a] of negative and positive hybridization controls and λ *Hind*III marker (made radioactive if possible) on a 1.0% (or less) agarose gel overnight.
3.	After electrophoresis is completed, stain the DNA with ethidium bromide and photograph the gel. (The gel can be trimmed at this stage to remove any unused lanes.)
4.	Denature the DNA by soaking the gel in 0.5 M NaOH, 0.5 M NaCl for 30 min at room temperature with gentle shaking.
5.	Rinse the gel with H_2O and neutralize in 0.5 M Tris-HCl (pH 8.0), 1.5 M NaCl for 30 min at room temperature with gentle shaking.
6.	Place the gel on two sheets of Whatman 3MM paper[b] and transfer to a gel dryer (e.g. Biorad, Model 1125B). Overlap the gel with cling film or Saranwrap and cover this with only the red neoprene rubber sheet which is part of the gel dryer.
7.	Dry the gel under vacuum initially without heat. When the gel is almost dry (flat), set the heater on 60°C and continue drying the gel under vacuum at 60°C for another hour. Release the vacuum, the gel should be a thin film[c] on the Whatman paper and can be stored indefinitely, at room temperature, until needed.

Variation

1.	If hybridization is to be done on N/C membrane, then DNA is transferred to N/C by Southern blot and baked after step 5.
2.	It is also possible to dry the gel after step 3 before denaturation and neutralization. In this case the dried gel is denatured and neutralized for 10 min each just prior to hybridization.

[a]Single-copy gene equivalent of 10 µg genomic DNA for cloned β-globin gene in pBR322 is 15 pg.
[b]The gel can be labelled at this stage if it is dried over a pencil written mark on the Whatman paper. This leaves an imprint on the dried gel.
[c]Make sure the gel is completely dry. If the Whatman paper feels damp, continue drying for another 30 min or so.

Table 2. Radiolabelling of oligonucleotides.

A.	5' ³²P-end labelling

1. Add in the following order:
    15 pmol oligonucleotide[a] (~ 0.1 μg for 19 mer)
    H₂O to bring total reaction volume to 10 μl
    1 μl 10 × kinase buffer[b]
    30−40 pmol [γ-³²P]ATP[c]
    Mix
2. Add 4 units of T₄ polynucleotide kinase. Mix and incubate at 37°C for 30 min.
3. Add 10 μl loading buffer[d]. Mix and leave in ice ready for separation.

B.   Labelling by 3' primer extension

(1) For phosphorylation of template a stock of phosphorylated template is prepared as follows.
    (i) Add in the following order:
        640 pmol oligonucleotide (~ 4 μg for 19 mer)
        H₂O to bring total reaction volume to 100 μl
        10 μl 10 × template buffer[e]
    (ii) Add 20 units of T₄ polynucleotide kinase. Mix and incubate for 3 h at 37°C. Heat the reaction tp 90°C for 10 min to inactivate the enzyme.

(2) For probe synthesis:
    (i) For the primer extension reaction dry down 15 pmol of each of the [α-³²P]dNTPs (highest specific activity available) in 0.3 ml Wheaton Micro Products glass vials and add in the following order:
        0.625 μl template oligonucleotide (from above 4 pmol)
        13.5 pmol primer oligonucleotide
        H₂O to bring total reaction volume to 5 μl
        1 μl 5 × extension buffer[f]
    (ii) Leave on ice to bring the reaction to 0°C. Add 3 units DNA polymerase I (Klenow). Mix and incubate at 0°C for 3 h.
    (iii) Add 5 μl of gel loading buffer[d]

---

[a]Determination of oligonucleotide concentration. Like other nucleic acids, oligonucleotides are measured spectrophotometrically. Unlike other nucleic acids, however, the base composition of different synthetic sequences can vary widely, making it difficult to make an accurate determination of concentration using an average extinction coefficient. In order to determine the concentration of an oligonucleotide solution, first calculate the molar extinction coefficient at 260 nm by summing the contribution of each nucleotide as follows: G: 12 010, A: 15 200, T: 8400 and C: 7050. This calculated number can then be used to determine the molar concentration of the oligonucleotide solution after measurement of the absorbance of the solution at 270 nm. For example: a 19-mer with five Gs, four As, five Cs and five Ts would have a molar extinction coefficient of 198 100 at 260 nm which is equivalent to 1 M/litre of the oligonucleotide solution.
i.e. at A_{260} 198 100 ≡ 1 M/l

$$1.0 \quad \equiv 5 \ \mu M/l$$

or 5 pmol/μl

Therefore, for this 19-mer with 1.0 OD/ml at A_{260}, we need 3.0 μl for 15 pmol of oligonucleotide probe. Oligonucleotides should be stored as frozen concentrated stock solutions in TE buffer (10 mM Tris-HCl pH 8.0, 1 mM EDTA) or as dried powders. The stock solutions are stable for several months or years.
[b]10 × kinase buffer is 670 mM Tris-HCl pH 8, 100 mM MgCl₂, 100 mM dithiothreitol (DTT).
[c]Two types of [γ-³²P]ATP are available: 1CN (crude) ~ 7000 Ci/mmol, Amersham PB15068 ~ 3000 Ci/mmol. For Amersham [γ-³²P]ATP PB15068, use 1.0 μl (equivalent to 50 pmol). If the volume of [γ-³²P]ATP is too high, dry it down and re-dissolve in 2 μl H₂O.
[d]Loading buffer is 0.05% xylene cyanol, 0.05% bromophenol blue, 20 mM Tris-HCl pH 7.5, 1 mM EDTA, 8 M urea.
[e]10 × template buffer is 300 μM ATP, 500 mM Tris-HCl, pH 9.0, 100 mM MgCl₂, 100 mM DTT, 500 μg/ml bovine serum albumin.
[f]5 × extension buffer is 125 mM Tris-HCl pH 7.5, 250 mM NaCl, 30 mM magnesium acetate.

4. TECHNICAL DETAILS

A typical protocol for oligonucleotide hybridization to DNA immobilized in dried agarose gel is summarized in *Tables 1—4*.

4.1 **General hints**

A number of general points relevant to many of the procedures are given below.

(i)   Make sure your DNA is completely digested. An indication of the completeness of digestion is the presence of low molecular weight cross-hybridizing bands which varies with the oligonucleotide probe. Comparison of the intensity of the cross-hybridizing band with that of the desired band gives an indication of the genotype of the individual.

(ii)   Because of the presence of cross-hybridizing bands it is important to include a DNA size marker, e.g. λ *Hin*dIII.

(iii)   Background hybridization can be a problem. 'Spotty' or 'measles' type background is usually due to probe contamination with unincorporated $[\gamma\text{-}^{32}P]ATP$ or to undissolved bits of agarose. Try filtering the agarose through a 0.8 μM Millipore nitrocellulose filter after boiling. 'Blotchy' type background is usually due to poor washing. Continue the room temperature wash following the 'hot' wash for a few hours if necessary.

(iv)   Sometimes it is desirable to locate fragments of more than 4 kb in size. To reduce the non-specific high molecular weight smearing, digest DNA with a second

Table 3. Separation of labelled oligonucleotide by gel electrophoresis.

1.	Cast a preparative 15% polyacrylamide gel (acrylamide:bis-acrylamide = 29:1) of 0.8—1.0 mm thickness in 7 M urea and 1 × TBE[a].
2.	Pre-electrophorese the gel at 25 W for 30 min to 1 h.
3.	Load the oligonucleotide samples and electrophorese at 25 W until the bromophenol blue (BPB) is at the bottom of the gel.
4.	At the end of the run, detach the plates from the tank, lay the gel sandwiched between the two glass plates flat on the bench. Lift up a corner of the upper glass plate, leaving the gel attached to the lower plate[b]. Remove the spacers.
5.	Cover the gel with cling wrap as smoothly as you can. Bind the two vertical sides of the gel with tape.
6.	Make radioactive markers asymmetrically on the tape. Expose the gel to a fast X-ray film (e.g. Kodak XAR-5) for a few minutes in a cassette and develop the film. Alternatively, place an X-ray film over the gel and pierce the film over the tape several times with a needle. These needle points act as markers for alignment of the film to the gel.
7.	Locate the labelled oligonucleotide by autoradiography and cut out the labelled bands on the X-ray films. By superimposing the X-ray film on the gel with the aid of the markers, excise the gel fragments containing the labelled probe. Check with Geiger counter to make sure that the correct gel fragments have been excised. Alternatively, check by re-exposing the gel to another X-ray film.
8.	Crush the gel slices and suspend in 10 mM Tris-HCl pH 7.5, 1 mM EDTA overnight at 37°C[c] to elute the labelled oligonucleotide.
9.	Centrifuge for 5 min and transfer the supernatant to a fresh tube.
10.	5 μl of supernatant is then counted in 5 ml of scintillation fluid.

[a]1 × TBE is Tris 10.8 g/l, boric acid 5.5 g/l, EDTA 0.95 g/l.
[b]Siliconization of the upper plate makes the operation easier.
[c]Gel slices can be incubated at 56°C for 3 h to hasten elution of probe.

Table 4. Hybridization and washing.

1.	Remove the dried gel from the paper backing by floating it on a shallow pan of water. The gel, which is now like a piece of cellophane, will float off the paper after a couple of minutes of gentle shaking.
2.	Slip the gel into a polythene bag sealed on three sides.
3.	No pre-hybridization is required for dried gels.
4.	Hybridize the gel for a minimum of 2 h at the appropriate temperature (5°C below calculated Td)[a] with 2×10^6 c.p.m./ml of 5' end-labelled oligonucleotide in $5 \times$ SSPE[b], 0.1% SDS, 100 μg/ml yeast tRNA[c].
5.	Remove the gel and wash 2×15 min in $6 \times$ SSC[d] at room temperature.
6.	Repeat the wash in $6 \times$ SSC at room temperature for 1 h.
7.	Wash for $1-2$ min in $6 \times$ SSC at the hybridization temperature.
8.	Repeat the room temperature wash in $6 \times$ SSC for $1-2$ h.
9.	Dry the gel between two sheets of 3MM Whatman paper and check the background with Geiger counter. If satisfactory (<2 c.p.m.) wrap the gel in cling film and autoradiograph with Kodak XAR-5 film between two intensifying screens (Cronex Lightning Plus) at -70°C overnight.
10.	Repeat steps 7 and 8 as necessary to obtain selectivity of hybridization. It is therefore necessary to always to include negative and positive hybridization controls.

Note: gels can be re-hybridized with a different probe after elution of the previous probe by denaturing and neutralizing the gel as in steps 4 and 5, *Table 1*, but in this case the incubation is reduced to 10 min each. Gels may be stored in X-ray cassettes at -20°C for at least 6 months between hybridizations or stored re-dried on Whatman 3MM paper.

[a]See section 3.4.2.
[b]$1 \times$ SSPE is 180 mM NaCl, 10 mM NaH_2PO_4, 1 mM EDTA (pH 8).
[c]tRNA can be substituted by any other non-specific nucleic acid sequences, e.g. calf thymus or *E. coli* DNA, salmon sperm DNA or oligoribonucleotides.
[d]$1 \times$ SSC is standard sodium citrate, 0.15 M NaCl, 0.015 M trisodium citrate, pH 7.0.

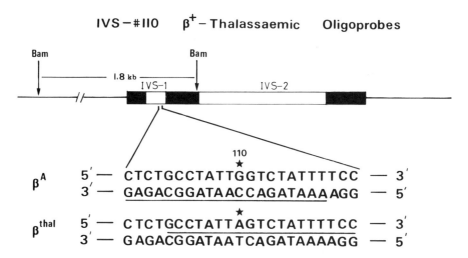

Figure 3. Preparation of synthetic oligonucleotide probes for the direct detection of the IVS1-110 β^+-thalass-aemic mutant. The β-globin gene is depicted at the top with its three coding blocks (solid) and two intervening sequences (IVS-1 and IVS-2). Below, the normal DNA sequence is depicted with the single base substitution of G to A at position 110 of IVS-1. The β^A probe corresponds to the non-coding sequence (underlined) of the normal β-globin gene and the β^{thal} probe corresponds to the coding sequence of the mutant gene. The probes were designed to avoid a $G-T$ mismatch.

45

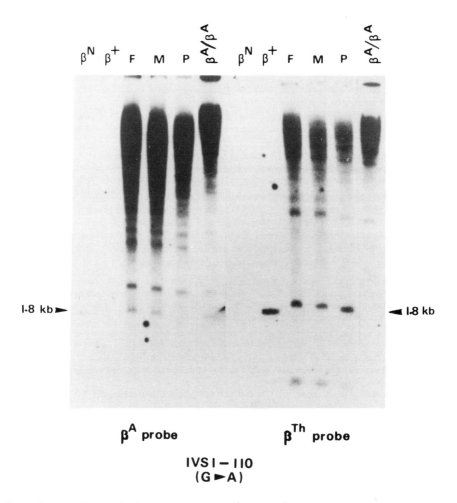

Figure 4. Autoradiogram of a family study using the IVS1-110 β^+ oligonucleotide probes. Hybridization was with β^A and β^{thal} (β^{th}) probes. Lane β^N = normal β plasmid DNA; β^+ = IVSI-110 β^+ plasmid DNA; F = father; M = mother; P = child; β^A/β^A = normal genomic DNA. Sequences of the β^A probe was 5'-AAATAGACCAATAGGCAGAG-3' and the βth probe was 5'-GCCTATTAGTCTATTTTCC-3'.

enzyme (as discussed in Section 3.1) and reduce the concentration of the agarose gel to 0.5% or 0.6%.

(v)   Poor hybridization signal can be caused by
(a) low specific activity of the probe;
(b) extremely high specific activity of the 5' ^{32}P end-labelled oligonucleotide leading to radiolysis and dilution of labelled oligonucleotide with unlabelled oligonucleotide;
(c) poor purification of the probe.

(vi)   No hybridization signal. Check the sequence of the oligonucleotide!

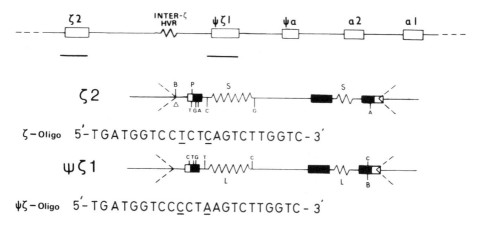

ζ-Oligo 5´-TGATGGTCC**T**CT**C**AGTCTTGGTC-3´

ψζ-Oligo 5´-TGATGGTCCC**C**TA**A**GTCTTGGTC-3´

Figure 5. Preparation of synthetic oligonucleotide probes to differentiate the ς and ψς-globin genes. The α-globin gene cluster is depicted above with the regions of homology between the ς2 and the ψς1 genes underlined. Below, the ς2 and the ψς1 globin genes are depicted with the six single base differences indicated. One of these, a G to T transversion in codon 6, introduces an inactivating amber mutation in the ς1 gene. Two nucleotides away is another single base change (A to G) in codon 7. The 'ς-oligo' probe corresponds to the zeta 23-nucleotide sequence and the 'ψς-oligo' corresponds to the pseudo-zeta 23-nucleotide sequence. The probes were designed to correspond to the non-coding sequence.

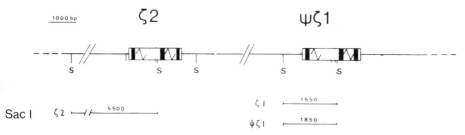

Figure 6. *Sac*I map of the zeta-like globin genes. The upstream ς globin gene is always associated with a 5.5-kb *Sac*I allele while the downstream gene can be associated with a 1.55- or 1.85-kb *Sac*I allele.

5. PRACTICAL APPLICATIONS

In this section we illustrate how synthetic oligonucleotides can be used to detect point mutations in the human genome.

5.1 Detection of the IVS1-110 β⁺ thalassaemia mutation

This is the most common form of β-thalassaemia in the Mediterranean region and results from a single nucleotide substitution (G→A) at position 110 of the first intervening sequence (IVS1) of the β-globin gene (29). This particular mutation is not directly detectable by restriction enzyme analysis. *Figure 3* shows the β-globin gene, the point mutation is contained in a *Bam*HI 1.8-kb fragment. To detect this point mutation two 19-base oligonucleotides were synthesized: one completely homologous to the normal coding β-globin gene sequence (β^A probe), the other to the thalassaemic non-coding β-globin gene sequence (β^thal probe) at a position around IVS1-110. The oligonucleotides were designed to avoid a G−T mismatch; β^A probe forms a C−A mismatch at the mutation

Synthetic oligonucleotides as hybridization probes

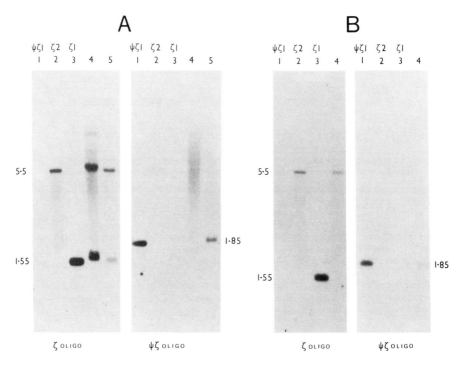

Figure 7. Oligonucleotide analysis of the zeta and pseudo-zeta globin genes. Oligonucleotide analysis of chromosomes with the 1.85- and 1.55-kb *Sac*I alleles. **Lanes 1, 2, 3** show the cloned DNA controls of known sequence. **Lane 1** = pBRs, a cloned 1.85-kb *Sac*I ψs1 allele; **lane 2** = pSVOD *Bam* 5.9, a cloned s2 *Sac*I 5.5 allele; **lane 3** = pαJs, a cloned 1.55-kb *Sac*I allele. **A: lane 4** = homozygote for the 1.55-kb *Sac*I alleleˊ **Lane 5** = heterozygote for the 1.55- and 1.85-kb *Sac*I alleles. **B: lane 4** = homozygote for the 1.85-kᴗ *Sac*I allele.

site with the β-thalassaemic DNA sequence while β^{thal} probe forms an A−C mismatch with the normal β-globin DNA sequence. *Figure 4* illustrates the results of a family study; father (F) and mother (M) are heterozygous while the child (P) is homozygous for β-thalassaemia. Both β^A and β^{thal} probes hybridized to DNA from father and mother who are therefore heterozygous for the IVS1-110 β^+ mutation. As expected, DNA from the child hybridized only to the β^{thal} probe. High molecular weight non-specific hybridization was observed with genomic DNAs but the *Bam*HI 1.8-kb fragment containing the mutation was clearly discernible. Low molecular weight cross-hybridizing bands were also seen with both the β^A and β^{thal} probes for the IVS1-110 β^+ mutant.

5.2 Differentiation of the zeta and ψ-zeta globin gene sequence

Sequence analysis has shown that the difference between a s and ψs gene include six point mutations and variation in the hypervariable regions (HVR) in introns I and II (*Figure 5*) (30). One of the six point mutations, a G to T transversion in codon 6, introduces an inactivating amber mutation in the ψs gene. Genomic mapping showed that whereas the upstream gene was always contained within a 5.5-kb *Sac*I s-specific fragment, the size of the *Sac*I fragment (*Figure 6*) containing the downstream gene was polymorphic, the majority of alleles being either 1.55 kb or 1.85 kb. Genomic mapp-

48

ing suggests that the downstream gene associated with the 1.85-kb *Sac*I fragment was ψs-like while that associated with the 1.55-kb *Sac*I fragment was s-like. The crucial difference which would define the ψs gene would be the inactivating mutation in codon 6 and this is not directly detectable by restriction enzyme analysis. To define this change, two 23-base long oligonucleotides were synthesized; one, the s-oligo, was completely homologous to the s-sequence and the other, ψs-oligo, was completely homologous to the ψs-sequence in the region of the amber mutation. The two oligonucleotide probes differ at two positions, representing the single base changes in codons 6 and 7 of exon 1.

We would like to point out a few relevant modifications in this application.

(i)   The two single base differences allow a longer oligonucleotide to be used, thus increasing hybridization specificity.

(ii)   In addition to *Sac*I, genomic DNA was digested with the enzyme *Hin*dIII which cut outside the *Sac*I fragments containing the s or ψs sequences to reduce the high molecular weight non-specific hybridization.

(iii)   The DNA fragments were electrophoresed on a 0.7% agarose gel again to reduce the non-specific high molecular weight hybridization.

Figure 7 shows that the s-oligo hybridized to 5.5-kb and 1.55-kb *Sac*I fragments while the ψs-oligo hybridized to the 1.85-kb fragment. Further analysis of eight populations (31) showed that the 5.5-kb and 1.55-kb *Sac*I fragments are always associated with zeta sequence while the 1.85-kb *Sac*I fragment is associated with a ψ-zeta sequence.

6. CONCLUSIONS

The technique of synthetic oligonucleotide hybridization has now proven indispensable for the detection of point mutations. However, there are a few limitations to this approach for prenatal diagnosis and carrier detection of genetic diseases. Unlike diagnosis by linkage analysis to restriction fragment length polymorphisms, the exact sequence of the normal and mutant gene must be known. There will be a spectrum of mutations causing the same disease phenotype and to cover all the mutations, a battery of oligonucleotide probes would be needed (7). Hence synthetic oligoprobes will not be so useful for those disorders which frequently arise from new mutations.

7. ACKNOWLEDGEMENTS

We thank Liz Gunson for typing the manuscript and Drs Sarah E.Ball, John Clegg and Kathryn Robson for helpful discussions.

8. REFERENCES

1. Antonarakis,S.E., Kazazian,H.H., Jr. and Orkin,S.H. (1985) *Hum. Genet.,* **69**, 1.
2. Wallace,R.B., Shaffer,J., Murphy,R.F., Bonner,J., Hirose,T. and Itakura,K. (1979) *Nucleic Acids Res.,* **6**, 3543.
3. Thomas,C.A., Jr. (1966) *Prog. Nucleic Acid Res. Mol. Biol.,* **5**, 315.
4. Conner,B.J., Reyes,A.A., Morin,C., Itakura,K., Teplitz,R.L. and Wallace,R.B. (1983) *Proc. Natl. Acad. Sci. USA,* **80**, 278.
5. Orkin,S.H., Markham,A.F. and Kazazian,H.H., Jr. (1983) *J. Clin. Invest.,* **71**, 775.
6. Pirastu,M., Kan,Y.W., Cao,A., Conner,B.J., Teplitz,R.L. and Wallace,R.B. (1983) *N. Engl. J. Med.,* **309**, 284.

7. Thein,S.L., Wainscoat,J.S., Old,J.M., Sampietro,M., Fiorelli,G., Wallace,R.B. and Weatherall,D.J. (1985) *Lancet,* **ii,** 345.
8. Kidd,V.J., Wallace,R.B., Itakura,K. and Woo,S.L.C. (1983) *Nature,* **304,** 230.
9. Bos,J.L., Toksoz,D., Marshall,C.J., Verlaan-de Vries,M., Veeneman,G.H., van der Eb,A.J., van Boom,J.H., Janssen,J.W.G. and Steenvoorden,A.C.M. (1985) *Nature,* **315,** 726.
10. Itakura,K., Rossi,J.J. and Wallace,R.B. (1984) *Annu. Rev. Biochem.,* **53,** 323.
11. Smith,M. (1983) In *Methods of DNA and RNA Sequencing,* Weissman,S.M. (ed.), Praeger, New York, p. 23.
12. Wallace,R.B., Schold,M., Johnson,M.J., Dembek,P. and Itakura,K. (1981) *Nucleic Acids Res.,* **9,** 3647.
13. Caruthers,M.H. (1985) *Science,* **230,** 281.
14. Bolton,E.T. and McCarthy,B.J. (1962) *Proc. Natl. Acad. Sci. USA,* **48,** 1390.
15. Suggs,S.V., Hirose,T., Miyake,T., Kawashima,E.H., Johnson,M.J., Itakura,K. and Wallace,R.B. (1981) In *Developmental Biology using Purified Genes,* Brown,D. (ed.), Academic Press, New York, p. 683.
16. Suggs,S.V., Wallace,R.B., Hirose,T., Kawashima,E.H. and Itakura,K. (1981) *Proc. Natl. Acad. Sci. USA,* **78,** 6613.
17. Wood,W.J., Gitschier,J., Lasky,L.A. and Lawn,R.M. (1985) *Proc. Natl. Acad. Sci. USA,* **82,** 1585.
18. Alwine,J.C., Kemp,D.J. and Stark,G.R. (1977) *Proc. Natl. Acad. Sci. USA,* **74,** 5350.
19. Wetmur,J.G. and Davidson,N. (1968) *J. Mol. Biol.,* **31,** 349.
20. Wahl,G.M., Stern,M. and Stark,G.R. (1979) *Proc. Natl. Acad. Sci. USA,* **76,** 3683.
21. Nei,M. and Li,W.H. (1979) *Proc. Natl. Acad. Sci. USA,* **76,** 5269.
22. Edge,M.D., Greene,A.R., Heathcliffe,G.R., Meacok,P.A., Schuch,W., Scanlon,D.B., Atkinson,T.C., Newton,C.R. and Markham,A.F. (1981) *Nature,* **292,** 756.
23. Wallace,R.B., Johnson,M.J., Hirose,T., Miyake,T., Kawashima,E.H. and Itakura,K. (1981) *Nucleic Acids Res.,* **9,** 879.
24. Southern,E.M. (1975) *J. Mol. Biol.,* **98,** 503.
25. Studencki,A.B. and Wallace,R.B. (1984) *DNA,* **3,** 7.
26. Sgaramella,V. and Khorana,H.G. (1972) *J. Mol. Biol.,* **72,** 127.
27. Bos,J.L., Verlaan-de Vries,M., Jansen,A.M., Veeneman,G.H., van Boom,J.H. and van der Eb,A.J. (1984) *Nucleic Acids Res.,* **12,** 9155.
28. Murasugi,A. and Wallace,R.B. (1984) *DNA,* **3,** 269.
29. Kazazian,H.H., Jr., Orkin,S.H., Markham,A.F., Chapman,C.R., Youssoufian,H. and Waber,P.G. (1984) *Nature,* **310,** 152.
30. Proudfoot,N.J., Gil,A. and Maniatis,T. (1982) *Cell,* **31,** 553.
31. Hill,A.V.S., Nicholls,R.D., Thein,S.L. and Higgs,D.R. (1985) *Cell,* **42,** 809.

CHAPTER 4

Alternative methods of gene diagnosis

J.LESLEY WOODHEAD, RACHEL FALLON, HERMIA FIGUEIREDO, JANE LANGDALE and ALAN D.B.MALCOLM

1. INTRODUCTION

A growing number of genetic diseases has now been attributed to a particular change in DNA sequence. There are single base pair changes which sometimes result in the deletion or addition of a site for a particular restriction enzyme (e.g. sickle cell anaemia). Sometimes the restriction enzyme site is not directly associated with the disease, but is closely linked, such that the change in restriction fragment length can be used for diagnosis. These are known as restriction fragment length polymorphisms (RFLP). Other changes include the deletion of large fragments of DNA and also interchromosomal rearrangements.

Thus both carrier detection and diagnosis of patients may now be performed using this information. This may even be performed antenatally. However, the methods involved are very labour intensive, involve the use of ^{32}P-labelled DNA (which is costly and has a short half-life) and cannot easily be automated (see Chapter 1 in this book). Random screening of a large population for an allele which occurs at a frequency as high as 1 in 50 (e.g. PKU) is not feasible as a present technology. We will describe in this chapter a method which is ideal for a routine laboratory and is easy to automate, unlike methods involving electrophoresis and Southern blotting.

1.1 Outline of basic method

The method involves a double (sandwich) hybridization where the sample under investigation may form a link between a labelled fragment and a second fragment covalently attached to a solid support. It can conveniently be illustrated by reference to sickle cell anaemia, which is caused by a single base pair mutation in the sixth codon of the human β-globin gene resulting in the loss of a *Dde*I (and *Mst*II) restriction enzyme recognition site. A restriction map of a 1.9-kb *Bam*HI fragment from the β-globin gene spanning the *Dde*I site is shown in *Figure 1*.

Two fragments are required, one of which, Fragment A, is attached to a resin. The other, Fragment B, is labelled and must be located on the opposite side of the mutation from Fragment A. In order to produce the sandwich, an additional fragment, C, which spans the gap between A and B, must be present. In our experiments the 341-bp *Hin*fI fragment was bound to S-500. The fragment B was a 201-bp *Mst*II fragment. These fragments were chosen so that they could be used with a *Dde*I digest of human DNA.

A sandwich hybridization can only form if the DNA under test is not cleaved by

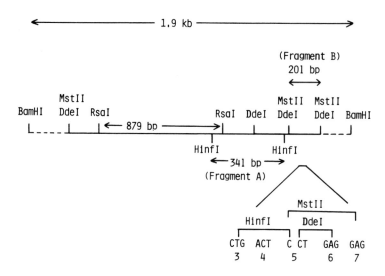

Figure 1. Partial restriction map for *Dde*I, *Mst*II, *Hinf*I and *Rsa*I sites in the 1.9-kb β-globin insert of the plasmid HβF-5. The base sequences of the five codons around the mutation site (GAG at position 6 → GTG) is shown in full.

*Dde*I at the β6 position, i.e. if the patient carries one or two chromosomes with a sickle mutation. In a normal individual, the DNA will be cleaved at this site and a double hybrid cannot result.

2. COUPLING OF DNA TO RESIN

The recommended method is that of Seed (1), with modifications (2). Of the various resins tested including Sephadex G-50, Sephadex G-200, cellulose and several Sephacryls, the Sephacryls, especially S-500, gave the highest percentage of covalent coupling with the lowest percentage of non-covalent attachment (3). The method is described as for S-500.

2.1 To make 2-aminophenylthioether derivative of resin

This derivative will be stable in the dark at 4°C for up to 1 year in water.

(i)   Wash 20 g aliquots with distilled water, and transfer to a 50 ml plastic screw top tube.

(ii)   Add 20 ml of 1 M NaOH and 1.7 ml of 1,4-butanediol diglycidylether. Rotate slowly end-over-end at room temperature, overnight.

(iii)   Filter the resin using a Buchner funnel. Press out as much aqueous solution as possible using a spatula, before returning the moist cake to the tube.

(iv)   Add 23 ml of acetone and 2.86 ml of 2-aminothiophenol. Seal the bottle and rotate end-over-end overnight at room temperature.

(v)   Wash in a Buchner funnel (in a fume hood!) with successively 200 ml each of acetone, 0.1 M HCl, water, 0.1 M HCl and water again.

(vi)   Resuspend the 2-aminophenylthioether (APTE) derivative of the resin in water.

2.2 **Diazotization of APTE resin**

The APTE Sephacryl can be conveniently diazotized in 1 g aliquots as follows.

(i)   Wash 1 g in a sintered glass funnel with 30 ml of distilled water then resuspend in 1 ml of water + 3.33 ml of 1.8 M HCl.

(ii)   Keep on ice for 30 min.

(iii) Add 33 μl aliquots of freshly made 10 mg/ml sodium nitrite. Follow the progress of the reaction by the use of starch iodide paper. Leave about 7 min between additions of nitrite. The reaction will be complete when the starch iodide paper remains blue. Typically this stage will be reached when four aliquots have been added and about 30 min have elapsed.

(iv)   *Quickly* transfer resin to an ice-cold sintered glass filter funnel and wash with 50 ml of ice-cold water, and finally with about 5 ml of ice-cold 25 mM sodium phosphate, pH 6.0 and dimethylsulphoxide (DMSO) 20:80 (v/v).

(v)   The resin will turn a darker colour during this last washing step. As soon as the surface of the resin becomes dry put 500 mg of the resin into an Eppendorf tube and add 250 μl of DNA solution. This solution is prepared by dissolving the dried down DNA pellet in 50 μl of sodium phosphate, pH 8.0 and adding 200 μl of DMSO.

   Results have shown that coupling efficiency does not vary greatly over the range 140−562 pmol DNA per g resin; also that percentage coupling does not vary significantly with the size of the fragment from 201 to 2700 bp.

(vi)   Incubate the reaction mixture for 2 days at room temperature, rotating end-over-end throughout.

(vii) Pour into a sintered glass funnel and wash with water and then 0.4 M NaOH at 4°C. Finally wash with 100 ml of 10 mM Tris-HCl, pH 7.5, 1 mM EDTA at room temperature. Store at 4°C.

2.3 **Assay of DNA linked to resin**

Two methods may be used.

2.3.1 *Radiolabelling*

(i)   Incorporate a tracer amount of [^{32}P]kinase-labelled DNA into the reaction and count by Cerenkov counting.

(ii)   After the immobilization reaction and washing, count the sample again. It will thus be possible to measure the amount of DNA coupled.

2.3.2 *Micrococcal nuclease digestion*

Nuclease assays are carried out essentially as described (2).

(i)   Wash 50 mg aliquots of the resin with 0.1 M sodium borate, pH 8.8 and transfer to Eppendorf tubes.

(ii)   Resuspend each aliquot in 400 μl sodium borate, pH 8.8 and 15 μl of 0.1 M CaCl$_2$. Add *Staphylococcus aureus* nuclease to a final concentration of 300 U/ml and incubate at 37°C overnight.

(iii) Re-centrifuge. Calculate the amount of DNA released by the nuclease into the supernate by measuring its absorbance at 260 nm. 1 O.D. unit of native DNA is equivalent to 1.6 units of digested DNA as a consequence of the hyperchromic effect.

The radiolabelling method gives a higher estimate for coupling efficiency than does the micrococcal nuclease. Typically values obtained for the former method with S-500 are about 80%, whereas the second method gives a value of about 50%. The second value reflects the percentage of DNA which is accessible to nuclease, and has been found to give a more accurate estimation of the hybridization potential of the resin.

2.4 Stability

Once the DNA is bound to the resin it is relatively stable if stored at 4°C; at least 50% of the DNA remains bound after a 6-month period.

3. RADIOLABELLING OF DNA

There are three different methods for DNA labelling and the choice will depend upon the sensitivity of the assay required. Kinase labelling is least sensitive and oligolabelling produces probes of the highest specific activity.

3.1 Kinase labelling

This method involves labelling the 5' end of the DNA using T4 polynucleotide kinase. The 5' terminus of the DNA may need to be dephosphorylated first.

(i)   Add 1 unit of calf alkaline phosphatase to 0.5 μg of DNA in 100 μl of 50 mM Tris-HCl, pH 9, 1 mM $MgCl_2$, 0.1 mM $ZnCl_2$, 1 mM spermidine. Incubate for 30 min at 37°C.

(ii)   Add a second unit of calf alkaline phosphatase and continue to incubate for another 30 min.

(iii)   Inactivate the enzyme by the addition of EDTA to a concentration of 25 mM and continue the incubation at 65°C for 20 min.

(iv)   Extract twice with phenol and twice with chloroform.

(v)   Precipitate the aqueous phase with two volumes of ethanol.

(vi)   Resuspend the pellet in 50 μl of 50 mM Tris-HCl, pH 7.5, 10 mM $MgCl_2$, 10 mM 2-mercaptoethanol.

(vii)   Add $25-50$ μC [γ-^{32}P]ATP (3000 Ci/mmol) and two units of T4 polynucleotide kinase.

(viii) Incubate at 37°C for 15 min.

(ix)   Chase with 1 μM ATP and incubate for a further 15 min at 37°C.

(x)   Remove unincorporated nucleotides by gel filtration through Sephadex G-50. Make a small column (e.g. a Pasteur pipette plugged with glass wool), run the column in 3 × SSC, 0.1% SDS (1 × SSC is 0.15 M NaCl, 0.015 M Na citrate, pH 7.5). Collect 100 μl (2-drop) fractions and count (Cerenkov) in a scintillation counter. The kinase-labelled probe will be eluted first.

3.2 **Nick translation**

This method uses two enzymes: DNase I which introduces single-stranded nicks in the probe and DNA polymerase I which repairs the nicks. The enzymes may be purchased in the correct buffer and at the appropriate relative ratios in a 'nick translation' kit available from commercial suppliers such as Bethesda Research Laboratories and Amersham International. Each kit comes with full instructions.

(i) Label 0.5 μg of DNA as outlined with $25-50$ μCi $[\alpha\text{-}^{32}P]$dCTP, by incubating for 2.5 h at 15°C.

(ii) Separate the unincorporated nucleotides by gel filtration as described for kinase labelling.

3.3 **Oligolabelling**

This method (4) labels DNA to a very high specific activity. It involves denaturing the DNA and then using random hexadeoxynucleotide primers together with a Klenow fragment of DNA polymerase and all four nucleotides, one or more of which will be radiolabelled. Klenow fragment is the larger of the two produced when DNA polymerase I is cleaved by subtilisin. It retains the $5'-3'$ polymerase activity but has lost the $5'-3'$ exonuclease activity. This produces a radiolabelled DNA molecule complementary to the non-radioactive denatured DNA.

(i) Boil the DNA fragment for 10 min, cool on ice, then use immediately.

(ii) Carry out the labelling reaction at 19°C in 50 μl of 200 mM N-2-hydroxyethyl-piperazine N'-2-ethanesulphonic acid (Hepes), pH 6.6, 50 mM Tris-HCl, 5 mM MgCl$_2$, 10 mM 2-mercaptoethanol. Add between 10 and 40 ng DNA, 2 units of the Klenow fragment, 400 μg/ml of bovine serum albumin (BSA) and 0.25 OD$_{260}$ units of hexadeoxyribonucleotides. Add non-radioactive deoxyribonucleotide triphosphates to a concentration of 20 μM each and 50 μCi $\alpha\text{-}^{32}$P-labelled deoxyribonucleotide.

(iii) After overnight incubation, separate precursor nucleotide triphosphates from the labelled DNA by gel filtration (as described previously).

A kit is also now available for carrying out this labelling reaction (Amersham International).

4. PREPARATION OF DNA FRAGMENTS FOR LINKING TO THE RESIN

The optimal input DNA concentration for linking to S-500 is 140 pmol/g resin. There is no significant effect of varying the fragment size over the range $200-3000$ bp. Thus considering the 341-bp fragment, 5' to the β-sickle mutation: molecular weight = 2.25×10^5. Hence 140 pmol is 31.5 μg/g of resin.

First calculate the amount of plasmid DNA which must be digested to generate the required amount of fragment, bearing in mind that methods used for extracting DNA from agarose or polyacrylamide gels give yields significantly less than 100% (between 30 and 50% is quite respectable).

(i) Digest the plasmid DNA containing the appropriate fragment with restriction enzyme, under conditions specified by the supplier of the enzyme.

(ii)   Separate the fragments by electrophoresis on agarose gel, between 1 and 2% depending upon the fragment size. 1% if the fragment is greater than 1 kb, 2% if the fragment is less than 0.5 kb.

(iii)   Stain the gel in ethidium bromide (50 μg/l) for 20 min and excise the band containing the appropriate fragment by visualizing the gel under u.v. light.

(iv)   Take the slice of agarose and drop gently into a dialysis bag full of electrophoresis buffer.

(v)   Remove most of the electrophoresis buffer and seal the bag.

(vi)   Lay the dialysis bag in an electrophoresis tank parallel to the electrodes. Turn on the power at 140 V for about 30 min, after which time the DNA will have moved from the agarose gel into the dialysis bag.

(vii)   Remove the gel slice from the dialysis bag and return the bag to the tank in the same orientation as before.

(viii)   Reverse the current for 2 min so that any DNA stuck on the dialysis bag will be dislodged.

(ix)   Remove the electrophoresis buffer from the dialysis bag and wash out the bag thoroughly.

(x)   Extract the DNA solution three times with water-saturated butan-1-ol to remove ethidium bromide. Follow this with two phenol and then two chloroform extractions.

(xi)   Finally ethanol precipitate the DNA by adding 0.1 volumes of 3 M sodium acetate, pH 5 and two volumes of ethanol at $-70°C$ for 30 min. Centrifuge the precipitated DNA at 16 000 g for 15 min. Re-dissolve the pellet in TE buffer and measure the OD_{260} to estimate the yield.

This method is the one which has been found to give optical yields. Other available methods are described in Maniatis *et al.* (5).

5. PREPARATION AND DIGESTION OF HUMAN DNA

5.1 Preparation of DNA from blood

Sandwich hybridizations, especially when used to differentiate between heterozygote and homozygote states, must be carried out with DNA which is essentially undegraded prior to restriction enzyme digestion. Collect blood into 5 mM EDTA. This chelates ions which are required by various nucleases and prevents clotting. The DNA should either be prepared immediately or the blood stored at $-70°C$.

The method described here is essentially that described in ref. (6).

(i)   Mix each 10 ml blood sample with 90 ml of 0.3 M sucrose, 10 mM Tris-HCl, pH 7.5, 5 mM $MgCl_2$, 1% Triton X-100 at 4°C to lyse the cells.

(ii)   Pellet the nuclei by centrifugation at 16 000 g, 4°C for 10 min.

(iii)   Use a Pasteur pipette to resuspend the pellet in 4.5 ml of 0.075 M NaCl, 0.024 M EDTA, pH 8.0. Add the following: 125 μl of 10% (w/v) SDS, 100 μl of proteinase K (10 mg/ml), 150 μl of water. Incubate at 55°C for 2 h.

(iv)   Extract three times in an equal volume of phenol (previously equilibrated with 20 mM Tris-HCl, pH 8). Centrifuging between extractions is performed at 7000 g for 5 min. This is followed by two extractions with an equal volume of chloroform/isoamyl alcohol (24:1).

(v)   Precipitate the DNA from the aqueous phase by the addition of 0.1 volumes of 3 M sodium acetate, pH 8.0 and two volumes of ethanol at room temperature.

(vi)   Remove the high molecular weight blob of DNA on the end of a bent Pasteur pipette and allow to dry.

(vii)   Dissolve in 10 mM Tris-HCl, pH 7.5, 1 mM EDTA, by rotating gently on a wheel at 4°C.

(viii) Calculate the amount of DNA by measuring OD_{260}. A 50 μg/ml solution will have an OD_{260} of 1, when measured in a 10 mm pathlength cuvette. If the OD_{260}/OD_{280} is less than 1.75, it should be phenol extracted again to remove contaminating protein. If this is not done it may be difficult to obtain a complete digestion with a restriction enzyme.

The expected yield from 10 ml of blood varies between 100 μg and 400 μg. Increased lymphocyte counts consequent upon infection will result in improved yields.

5.2 Restriction digestion of human DNA

A complete restriction digestion of human DNA can usually be achieved by the addition of 5 units of enzyme per μg DNA and digesting overnight (16 h) at the recommended temperature for the particular enzyme, under the conditions specified by the manufacturer. However, since the sandwich hybridization method described here is dependent upon total digestion of the sample in order to discriminate between heterozygote and homozygote, trial experiments using different amounts of enzyme and or time should be carried out. The fragments can be separated on agarose and/or polyacrylamide gels, Southern blotted and probed with ^{32}P-labelled to probes to ascertain whether complete digestion has occurred at the site under investigation.

6. HYBRIDIZATION TO DNA IMMOBILIZED ON RESIN

It is first necessary to carry out a one-step hybridization with labelled probe of the same sequence as the DNA fragment linked to the column. This should be carried out in 1.5 ml screw cap Eppendorf tubes, rotating on a wheel in a fan-controlled incubator. This experiment will ascertain whether the DNA is linked in such a way as to be available for hybridization.

6.1 One-step hybridization

(i)   Incubate resin (use amount containing ~1 pmol of fragment) for 2 h in 1 ml of pre-hybridization buffer (40 mM Pipes, pH 6.5, 0.6 M NaCl, 1 mM EDTA, 0.1% w/v SDS and 250 μg/ml denatured, sonicated salmon sperm DNA at 65°C) (7) (to avoid high backgrounds the salmon sperm must be sonicated to 500 bp or less).

(ii)   Pellet the resin and remove the supernate.

(iii)   Hybridize with 20 fmol of denatured probe + 50 μl of the above buffer at 65°C for 1 h. The relatively short hybridization time suitable for fragments up to 3000 bp is due to the high probe concentration compared with hybridization on filters.

(iv)   Pellet the resin and wash three times for 10 min each at 65°C in 1 ml of the above buffer without salmon sperm DNA. Count the samples by Cerenkov counting in a scintillation counter.

It has been found that increasing the amount of immobilized DNA up to 100-fold excess over free DNA increases hybridization. The optimal concentration is about 50-fold for fragments between 200 and 3000 bp. Varying the amount of immobilized DNA from 50 to 220 pmol/g does not affect hybridization efficiency. The maximum efficiency is generally about 60%. This figure is calculated by setting up two controls, one with resin containing no DNA and the other in which labelled non-specific (e.g. calf thymus) DNA is used as a probe. These two controls generally give the same background reading. The percentage hybridization is given by:

$$\frac{(\text{Counts attached in experimental tube } - \text{ background counts})}{\text{Total counts possible}} \times \frac{100}{1}$$

6.2 Two-step sandwich hybridization

Optimal conditions for two-stage hybridization are as follows.

All hybridization should be carried out in the buffer used for one-step hybridizations. The addition of Denhardt's (8), dextran sulphate, or 1% glycine does not increase the hybridization efficiency (unlike hybridizations after Southern blotting). Absence of salmon sperm DNA was, however, found to increase the background 2-fold. It was also found to be important that this DNA is sonicated to 500 bp or less otherwise the background increases.

It is easier to carry out the development of the method using a specific restriction fragment as the middle part of the sandwich. The following protocol was found to work well for the detection of sickle cell anaemia. It should be noted, however, that there may be a problem if Fragments A and B are found to cross-hybridize. This has, in fact, been found to be a problem with the setting up of a sandwich assay for the detection of hepatitis B (9). Various pairs of fragments were shown to cross-hybridize in spite of having no detectable sequence homology. Before embarking on experiments involving linking a Fragment A on Sephacryl it is advisable to restrict the test DNA, separate the fragments on a gel, blot onto cellulose nitrate and hybridize with Fragment A and separately with B. There should be no cross-hybridization.

Figure 1 shows the appropriate fragments used in the sickle cell detection described here.

The Eppendorf tubes containing the resin should be rotated on a wheel throughout both pre-hybridization and hybridization.

(i)   Pre-hybridize the resin with 1 ml of the solution used in one-step hybridization, without the probe, at 65°C for 2 h. Use a 50-fold excess of immobilized DNA over sandwich DNA, although detection of a very few amol of sandwich DNA may necessitate greater than 50-fold excess since small amounts of resin are difficult to measure.

(ii)   Centrifuge and remove supernate. Add 50 µl of sandwich DNA and a 50-fold excess of labelled DNA. Hybridize at 65°C overnight or at least for a minimum of 8 h.

(iii)   Wash the resin three times at 10 min each in 1 ml of pre-hybridization solution without salmon sperm DNA.

We have found that hybridizations carried out at 37°C in 50% formamide took approximately 16 h to reach a maximum (cf. 8 h at 65°C without formamide). Adding the sandwich and the probe DNA sequentially does not affect the overall hybridization efficiency. The overall efficiency after correcting for non-specific attachment of probe DNA is approximately 28%, which implies about 53% at each individual hybridization step.

The sensitivity of the sandwich method is limited by the problem of non-specific hybridization of probe to resin which ultimately results in the size of the signal due to specific hybridization being not significantly different from background.

It has been found that by using oligolabelled DNA (high specific activity 6×10^7 d.p.m./pmol) as the probe, it is possible to detect as little as 10 amol (10^{-18} mol) of sandwich DNA. This is equivalent to a single copy sequence in 20 μg of total human DNA.

Attempts made to increase the sensitivity of the assay using larger free probe DNA (1200 bp) resulted in inconsistent results, which is thought to be due to the larger fragments becoming trapped non-specifically in the pores of the resin. It is possible that this problem may be overcome by the use of Sephacryl S-1000 which has an exclusion limit of 20 kb.

6.3 Sandwich hybridizations with human samples

Carry out the experiment in exactly the same way as previously described for two-step hybridizations. Using 20 μg of *totally* digested human DNA, 50 fmol of immobilized DNA fragment, and 0.5 fmol of oligolabelled probe, it is possible to differentiate between normal, heterozygotes and homozygotes. As noted before, problems may arise if the DNA sample is degraded, giving low results. In order to rule out this possibility every DNA sample can be checked for degradation by screening each sample for a gene which would be expected not to vary among the people under test, e.g. α-globin.

7. NON-RADIOACTIVE METHODS OF DNA DETECTION

For a method of gene detection to be suitable for routine diagnosis in a hospital laboratory it should ideally be amenable to automation, rapid, safe and inexpensive. The method described above fulfils the first two criteria adequately. However, the use of ^{32}P-labelled probe presents a potential safety problem and also means that the probe has short shelf life ($t\frac{1}{2} = 14.3$ days). A non-radioactively labelled probe would provide a satisfactory solution. We describe now the present range of methods available for the non-radioactive detection of DNA.

As yet no satisfactory results have been obtained using these probes for hybridization to immobilized DNA. The methods are satisfactory for DNA dotted or blotted onto cellulose nitrate filters. They fall into two categories. Either any enzyme can be cross-linked to the DNA directly, or the DNA can be modified in some way (e.g. by biotinylation) which enables subsequent detection by an enzyme-linked antibody.

7.1 Cross-linking of enzyme to DNA — the Renz method

The method which has been used in our laboratory for cross-linking horseradish peroxidase (HRP) to DNA is based on that described by Renz and Kurz (10). We are also developing a method which involves HRP linking to DNA via SPDP (Pharmacia), but this method is not yet ready for routine application and will not therefore be described here.

In the Renz method a protein is linked to a small positively-charged polymer. This modified protein is able to interact electrostatically with the DNA, thus facilitating high percentage cross-linking. The proteins used by Renz and Kurz are HRP or alkaline phosphatase. The small polymeric cation is polyethyleneimine G35 (mol. wt. ~ 1400) available from BASF, though as the authors point out, any amino-containing small molecular weight polymer would do, the histones for instance.

7.1.1 *Synthesis of polyethyleneimine conjugates (Solution A)*

(i)   Dissolve 20 mg of HRP (Grade I Boehringer) in 200 μl of 90 mM sodium phosphate, pH 6.0 in an Eppendorf tube.

(ii)   Make a fresh solution containing 30 mg of *p*-benzoquinone in 1 ml of ethanol, add 60 μl of this to the HRP solution.

(iii) Allow the mixture to react for 1 h in the dark at 37°C. For this use a rotating wheel in an oven or hot room. Cover the tube with aluminium foil.

(iv)   Remove non-reacted benzoquinone by gel filtration through Sephadex G-100, in a Pasteur pipette. This should be pre-equilibrated and run in 0.15 M NaCl. Two peaks will be seen: the first is a brown peroxidase peak followed by a yellow benzoquinone peak.

(v)   Combine the brown coloured fractions (~ 1.7 ml).

(vi)   Raise the pH by adding 180 μl of 1 M NaHCO$_3$ (freshly made) then add 2.7 μl (133 μg) of polyethyleneimine G35 solution.

(vii) Incubate the mixture for 20 h in the dark at 37°C, again rotating on a wheel.

(viii) Dialyze the solution against 5 mM phosphate, pH 6.8, with two changes of buffer over a 24 h period.

(ix)   The resultant *Solution A* may be stored at 4°C. No loss in activity will be observed during a 3 month period.

The cross-linking with alkaline phosphatase can be carried out in a similar way. Dialyze 3 mg of alkalkine phosphatase, 350 μl (from calf intestine) against 0.1 M sodium phosphate, pH 6.0. Carry out the cross-linking as with HRP, but adding 90 μl of the benzoquinone solution. Use a G-100 column to separate benzoquinone from alkaline phosphatase and to the pooled enzyme fractions add 100 μl of 1 M NaHCO$_3$ and 20 μg of polyethyleneimine. The final solution can also be stored at 4°C for several months without deterioration.

7.1.2 *Construction of the probe*

The probe can be constructed using any linear DNA molecule. It is cross-linked to the PEI enzyme conjugates as follows.

(i)   Denature 1 μg of DNA in 20 μl of 5 mM sodium phosphate, pH 6.8, by heating in a 100°C water bath for 3 min, and then plunging into a bath of solid CO_2 and ethanol.

(ii)   To the frozen pellet add 20 μl of Solution A, allow to thaw and then add 6 μl of a 5% (v/v) glutaraldehyde solution.

(iii)   Incubate at 37°C for 10 min.

(iv)   The probe may then be used directly for hybridization or the DNA−PEI−HRP conjugates can be separated from PEI−HRP as follows:

(v)   Add 28 μl of a 40% solution (w/v) polyethylene glycol 8000 (Sigma).

(vi)   Centrifuge for 6 min and dissolve sediments in 10 μl of 1.5 M L-glycine in 5 mM sodium phosphate, pH 6.8. This solution is now ready for hybridization.

7.2 Biotinylation of DNA by nick translation

Biotinylated nucleotides can be incorporated into DNA by the method of Langer *et al.* (11) using nick translation (see previous section). The biotin is linked covalently to the carbon 5 position of the pyrimidine ring through an allylamine linker arm of variable length. After hybridization one method for visualizing the hybridized probe is by allowing streptavidin peroxidase to bind to the DNA and then stain for peroxidase. This, and other methods, will now be described.

(i)   Add 1 μg of linear DNA to a solution containing 2.5 units of DNA polymerase I, 250 ng of DNase I, 250 nmol of $MgCl_2$, 500 ng of BSA, 1 nmol each of dATP, dTTP, dCTP and biotin-11-dUTP in 50 μl 50 mM Tris-HCl, pH 7.8.

(ii)   Incubate for 90 min at 15°C.

(iii)   Separate biotinylated DNA from free nucleotides by chromatography through Sephadex G-50. In order to detect biotinylated DNA, spot fractions onto cellulose nitrate and assay for biotin by the antibody method (11). The earlier eluting biotin-containing peak will contain the biotinylated DNA.

A greater degree of biotinylation can be achieved by the method of oligolabelling (see Section 3.3). However, there is considerable doubt as to whether the more highly substituted DNA does in fact hybridize as efficiently (12).

7.3 Hybridization of non-radioactive probes

Linear DNA is transferred to cellulose nitrate (Schleicher and Schull) by Southern blotting. The amounts of DNA which can be detected by each of these methods will be discussed later (Section 7.4).

7.3.1 *Hybridization of enzyme-labelled probe*

(i)   Soak filters in 10 × Denhardt's, 4 × SET (1 × SET is 0.15 M NaCl, 0.03 M Tris-HCl, pH 8.0, 1 mM EDTA) and 0.1% SDS for 1 h at 38°C.

(ii)   Transfer the filters to 20 μl of a pre-hybridization buffer containing 50% deionized formamide, 2 × Denhardt's, 4 × SET, 0.1% SDS and 30 μg/ml yeast tRNA (Boehringer) for 1 h at 38°C.

(iii)   Hybridize the filters overnight in 10 ml of pre-hybridization buffer, containing 500 ng/ml of enzyme-labelled probe and 6% PEG at 38°C.

(iv)   Wash the filters in two changes of 50% de-ionized formamide, 0.4% SDS and 0.5 × SSC at 38°C for 60 min followed by two washes of 2 × SSC at room temperature for 20 min.

(v)   Soak the filters in 0.1 M sodium phosphate, pH 8.0.

7.3.2 *Hybridization of biotion-labelled DNA*

(i)   Incubate the filters for 2 h at 65°C in 3 × SSC, 10 × Denhardt's, 200 μg/ml of salmon sperm DNA, 0.1% SDS, 0.1% sodium pyrophosphate.

(ii)   Transfer the filters to hybridization buffer, which is as previous buffer but also contains 10% dextran sulphate and 100 ng/ml of denatured biotinylated DNA probe. Incubate filters for 16 h at 65°C.

(iii)   Wash the filters twice in 2 × SSC, 0.1% SDS at room temperature. Wash twice more in 0.2 × SSC, 0.1% SDS, again at room temperature.

(iv)   Carry out two stringent washes in 0.16 × SSC, 0.1% SDS at 50°C for 15 min.

(v)   Rinse the filters briefly in 2 × SSC, 0.1% SDS at room temperature.

(vi)   Block the filters by incubating in 3% BSA in phosphate-buffered saline (PBS) for 20 min at 42°C.

Figure 2. Oxidation of luminol by hydrogen peroxide.

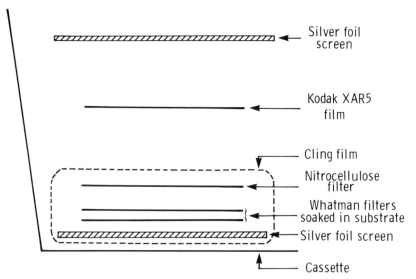

Figure 3. Diagram of the arrangement of filters, film and screens in an autoradiography cassette. The Whatman filters are dampened with substrate and placed on the screen, inside a cling film envelope. The nitrocellulose filter is gently placed on top of the Whatman filters, making sure that no air bubbles are present. Pre-flashed Kodak XAR5 film is placed on top, followed by another silver foil screen. The cassette is closed and left at room temperature for the appropriate exposure time.

Table 1. Sensitivity of detection of the plasmid βf5 immobilized on cellulose nitrate.

Type of probe used	Detection system		
	Luminol/luciferin luminescent assay	*o-dianisidine chromogenic assay*	*NBT/BCIP chromogenic assay*
Chemically-modified HRP-labelled βf5	13 amol	27 amol	—
Nick-translated biotion-labelled βf5	270 amol	27 amol	27 amol
Oligolabelled-biotinylated βf5	270 amol	27 amol	27 amol

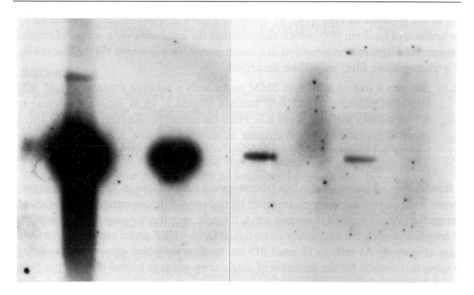

Figure 4. 10, 1, 0.1, 0.05, 0.01 ng of plasma βf5 DNA was Southern blotted onto cellulose nitrate. The filters were hybridized with 0.5 μg of βf5 DNA, labelled with peroxidase. The peroxidase was visualized by luminol and luciferin after a 30 min exposure to Kodak XAR5 film.

(vii)   Dry the filters at 80°C for 10 min.

(viii) Incubate the filters for 30 min with either streptavidin peroxidase complex (1:60) (Amersham International) in PBS, or with streptavidin followed by biotinylated polymer of alkaline phosphatase (BRL detection kit). Remove excess streptavidin: peroxidase by washing three times in PBS for 30 min.

Note: Full details for these procedures are not given here since very full instructions are given with the detection kit from BRL.

7.4 Detection of non-radiactive probe

7.4.1 Chromogenic detection

It has been found (12) that *o*-dianisidine is a sensitive substrate for peroxidase detection on cellulose nitrate. Tetramethylbenzidine [a sensitive substrate for HRP in solution (13)] does not detect the Renz probe filters and also binds to DNA itself, which may produce spurious results.

(i)   Incubate HRP-labelled filters in the dark with a solution containing (in 10 ml) 6 mg of *o*-dianiside (Sigma) in 2 ml of ethanol, 0.03% hydrogen peroxide,

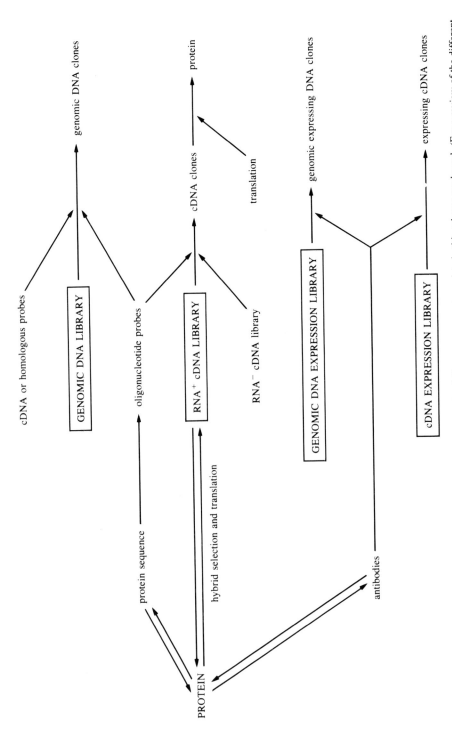

Figure 1. Flow chart for the isolation of cDNA and genomic DNA clones. The different start or entry points in this scheme are boxed. (For a review of the different cloning and screening procedures see ref. 1–3.)

3. MAPPING THE TRANSCRIPTIONAL UNIT

If we assume for illustrative purposes that we have either complete or partial genomic and cDNA clones for a gene containing three exons and two introns, we would have to analyse the following RNA polymerase II transcriptional unit; a primary transcript that is initiated at the first nucleotide of the first exon and terminated somewhere past the last nucleotide of the last exon. The primary transcript is processed to produce the mature mRNA at several positions; the introns are removed by a splicing process (11) and the 3′ end is formed by an endonucleolytic cleavage and polyadenylation (12). There are of course many exceptions to this general scheme, e.g. histone genes without introns or a poly(A) tail. A number of different techniques can be used to analyse the transcription unit:

(i)   Northern blots;
(ii)   cDNA genomic DNA comparison;
(iii)   R looping;
(iv)   nuclease protection experiments;
(v)   'transcription run-off' analysis.

Each of these techniques have their particular advantages and limitations.

3.1 Restriction map

The simplest method which also provides a basis for all further mapping of the transcriptional unit, is the construction of a restriction map using a number of different restriction enzymes (13). If both genomic and cDNA clones are available, a comparison of the two will give an immediate approximate indication of the localization of the exons and introns. This information is roughly confirmed by 'Southern blot' (14) analyses of the genomic DNA with the cDNA. This type of analysis originally led to the first proposal by Jeffreys and Flavell (15) that the β-globin gene contained at least one intron between two particular restriction sites. For our purpose, let us assume a gene, as shown in *Figure 2*. A genomic clone containing three exons and two introns plus the restriction sites A to E and a cDNA clone containing the sites B, C and D.

3.2 Northern blots

A second invaluable method used in transcription mapping is 'Northern' blotting (16). In this method the RNA is electrophoresed in denaturing gels and transferred to nitrocellulose (or other) filters and hybridized to the cloned cDNA or genomic DNA to determine the size of the mature mRNA and its precursors. For the gene illustrated in *Figure 2* the smallest (and usually most intensely) hybridizing band would be the mature polyadenylated mRNA containing exons I, II and III (i.e. the same as the cDNA). In addition, higher molecular weight RNAs could be detected which correspond to precursor RNAs, in our example exons I, II and III plus one or both of the introns. By using different probes, each of the exons and introns could be assigned in order (17). This method is very sensitive and can even be used to detect an intron in free linear and lariat form introns (18).

The combination of restriction maps and the use of several probes in Northern blots usually gives a fairly good global picture of the transcriptional unit, although any precise coordinates will not, as yet, have been established.

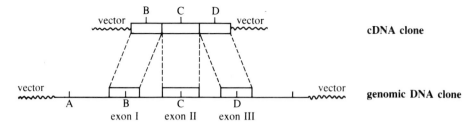

Figure 2. Structure of a theoretical eukaryotic gene and its DNA. The letters A to E indicate restriction enzyme sites.

3.3 'Run-on' transcription

The reverse procedure of the Northern blot described above is a Southern blot using labelled RNA. This procedure is particularly important to localize the termination of transcription which proceeds past the poly(A) addition site at the 3' end of the mRNA (19). This technique is based on *in vitro* transcription in isolated nuclei in the presence of radiolabelled ribonucleotides. Under these circumstances, very little new initiation or RNA synthesis takes place. Only RNA chains initiated *in vivo* are elongated by several hundred nucleotides (20) and only partial processing of completed chains occurs (21).

The labelled RNA is isolated and hybridized to Southern blotted or dot blotted restriction fragments of the cloned gene. The DNA fragments that are transcribed will hybridize and be visible on the autoradiograph. In the case of the mouse β-globin gene (*Figure 3*), the hybridization shows no signal for fragments upstream of the gene, an equal signal for fragments covering and directly downstream of the gene and a decreasing signal in further downstream fragments. From these results the authors concluded that transcription termination does not take place at a discrete site, but over an area of about 1 kb (22). Because this method is not sensitive enough to detect very short hybrids and because the length of the hybrid is not measured, the boundaries of the transcription unit can only be determined to within a few hundred base pairs (23).

3.4 **R looping**

A more visual localization of intron-exon is possible using electron microscopy (EM) and R looping (24). Because of the techniques and machinery involved, this technique will not be readily available everywhere and requires considerable EM experience. We will, therefore, not provide a lab protocol, but only refer to published work. It is, however, very informative and is definitely very useful when a gene with a large number of exons and introns has to be handled. Moreover, it will demonstrate whether within the limits of detection all the mRNA is accounted for in terms of cloned DNA, or whether the cloned gene is still incomplete. The method is based on the observation that DNA-RNA hybrids are of the A-type helix, whereas duplex DNA is in the B-type form. This difference in structure causes a different stability in different solvents. In formamide DNA-RNA hybrids are more stable, while in aqueous solutions duplex DNA is more stable (25,26). In order to form R loops, duplex DNA and RNA are hybridized in a formamide solution close to the melting temperature of the DNA duplex. Transient

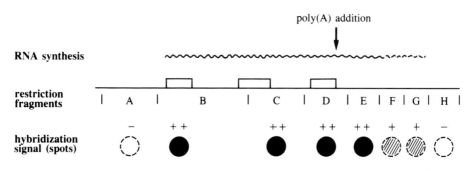

Figure 3. A theoretical 'run-on' hybridization. The restriction fragments A to H are spotted onto nitrocellulose filters and hybridized to 'run-on' labelled RNA + +, +, − indicate strong, weak and zero hybridization signals, respectively.

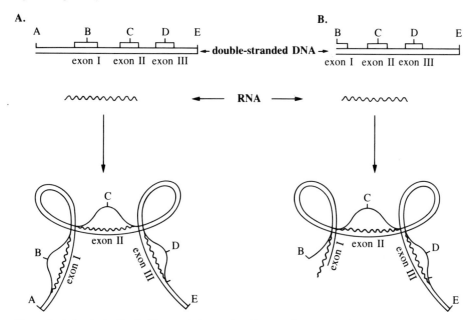

Figure 4. 'R-looping'. The double-stranded genomic DNA (A to E or B to E) is hybridized to RNA under R looping conditions.

single-stranded regions will hybridize to the complementary RNA and form stable hybrids, displacing the complementary DNA strand which is visible as a single strand (R) loop (*Figure 4A*). By using different restriction enzymes it is possible to position the transcriptional unit within about 100 bp. In our example we would expect the type of structure shown in *Figure 4A*, which was first observed for the globin and ovalbumin genes (17,27). Structures such as shown in *Figure 4B* would indicate that the DNA clones are incomplete. Alternatively, when the DNA clones are deliberately shortened (e.g. by cleavage at site B) the combination of *Figure 4A* and *4B* would map the transcript.

3.5 **Nuclease S1 protection and Southern blots**

The remainder of the techniques which we will discuss are all based on the same very basic hybridization techniques we have already mentioned, but are much more precise in their measurement and use of enzymatic reactions. The methods are mostly based on nuclease S1 protection experiments that were originally developed by Berk and Sharp (28) to map the transcripts of early adenovirus genes. Nuclease S1 from *Aspergillus oryzae* is an enzyme that degrades single-stranded DNA or RNA (29). Double-stranded DNA, RNA and DNA-RNA hybrids are resistant to degradation unless very large amounts of the enzyme are used. A similar enzyme is mung bean nuclease (30), although this enzyme will not cleave the DNA strand opposite a nick in a duplex, while nuclease S1 will. These enzymes can, therefore, be used to measure the size of a DNA-RNA hybrid by cleavage of the non-hybridized single-stranded nucleic acid. If we apply the technique to our example, we could expect the following (*Figure 5*). The RNA preparation which contains the primary transcript, processing intermediates and the mature mRNA is hybridized with a denatured genomic DNA fragment under high formamide conditions where DNA-DNA annealing is prevented. Several different hybrids will be formed. The primary transcript will hybridize to the DNA over its full length, whereas in the case of spliced mRNA or intermediates, hybrid molecules will be formed that contain loops of intron DNA. (The opposite would be obtained with

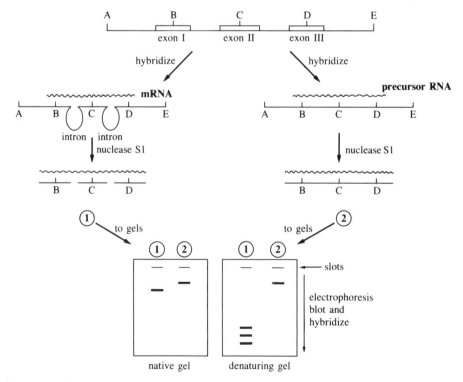

Figure 5. Nuclease S1 protection analysis on Southern blots. The genomic DNA (A to E) is hybridized to an RNA population containing processed mRNA and precursor RNA. The RNA-DNA hybrids are treated with nuclease S1 [(1) and (2)] and analysed on agarose gels.

cDNA, i.e. the precursor would be contained in a hybrid with RNA loops, while the mRNA would be present in a co-linear hybrid). The hybrids are then treated with nuclease S1, which destroys the single-stranded nucleic acid but leaves the hybrids intact. Consequently, the primary transcript will be reduced to a full length perfect duplex, by removal of the excess single-stranded DNA and RNA tails. The processed transcript will similarly be reduced to a hybrid with two nicks in the DNA at the positions where the intron DNA loops were removed by the nuclease S1. The two types of molecules can be distinguished by agarose gel electrophoresis under denaturing and non-denaturing conditions. The RNA will be destroyed by alkali in the denaturing gel and will still be present in the hybrid on the non-denaturing ('native') gel. The primary transcript will be the same full length fragment on both gels. The spliced transcript would become visible as a single band on the native gel and as three separated bands, each the size of the individual exons on the alkaline gel. Usually unlabelled DNA fragments are used in the hybridization to the RNA and the nuclease S1 protected fragments are only detected after Southern blotting of the gel and hybridization to labelled DNA probes from the same gene. This method has the advantage (over subsequent methods) that it can be used with long DNA fragments containing multiple exons and introns. In one experiment a fairly good picture of the transcriptional unit can be obtained. This is especially true when two dimensional electrophoresis is used, one dimension at neutral pH, the second dimension at alkaline pH, and when the blots are hybridized to different probes corresponding to different parts of the gene (31). The disadvantage (particularly for long fragments on agarose gels), is that the sizes are not absolutely precise, due to inaccuracies in the marker sizing and diffusion of the bands during the blotting procedure.

3.6 Nuclease S1 protection of end-labelled probes

Once the (approximate) position of the exon, or later when some restriction sites in an exon are known, end-labelled probes can be used for a very precise localization of exon and intron borders. The procedure is a variation of the Berk and Sharp method, but instead of using unlabelled probes, restriction fragments are used that are only label-led at the ends (32). For example, for our test gene we could use DNA probes from restriction sites A to B and B to C. The fragments can be labelled in two ways, either at the 5′ ends using polynucleotide kinase (33) or at the 3′ ends by 'filling in' or 'replacement' synthesis using DNA polymerase I (Klenow fragment) (34), T4 DNA polymerase (35) or reverse transcriptase (36). The labelled DNA fragment is subsequently denatured and hybridized to the RNA in high formamide concentrations. Higher sensitivity (almost always unnecessary), can be obtained by separating the individual strands of the DNA probe by polyacrylamide gel electrophoresis (37) prior to use. After hybridization, the samples are treated with nuclease S1 which will degrade all the single-stranded regions. The protected hybrids are subsequently denatured and electrophoresed on polyacrylamide gels in the presence of 6 M urea, using a sequence ladder of the same fragment as a very precise size marker (*Figure 6(i)*). In our example (*Figure 6(ii)*) the kinased AB fragment would measure the 5′ end initiation point of the mRNA. The kinased BC fragment would measure the splice acceptor site (fragment 3) of the first intron, whereas the 'filled in' fragment would measure the splice donor site of the first intron (fragment 4). The fragments 2 and 5 would not show up in the

Fine mapping of genes

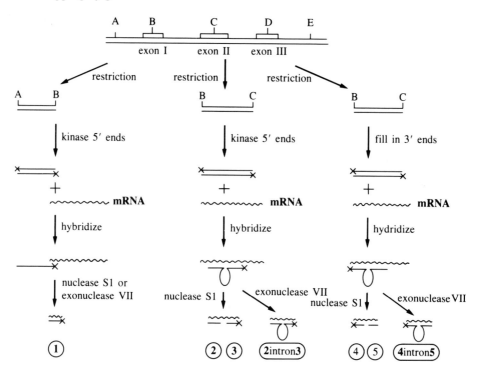

Figure 6. Nuclease S1 protection analysis with end labelled DNA probes. The genomic DNA fragments AD and BC are labelled at the 5′ or 3′ ends by 'kinase' or 'fill-in' reaction and hybridized to mRNA. The RNA-DNA hybrids are treated wtih nuclease S1 or exonuclease VII.

analysis because they are not labelled. *Figures 7A and B* are an example of a 5′ and 3′ end analysis of the mRNA transcribed off the human β-globin gene. The AB 5′ end probe of the example is represented by a kinased *Mbo*II-*Cvn*I restriction fragment. For the 3′ end analysis a 'filled in' *Eco*RI-*Msp*I fragment was used. A G+A sequence ladder provides a very precise measurement of the mRNA 5′ end in *Figure 7A*. It is obvious that this is a very precise method because it provides a border at an exact distance from a known restriction site. The disadvantage is that multiple probes have to be used to map each border of all the exons; in our example, at least four fragments for six S1 assays (AB, BC2×, CD2× and DE). Moreover, it should be remembered that this technique has to be supplemented with at least one other technique such as primer extension when the number of exons is unknown (see below at primer extension).

3.7 Exonuclease VII

A very useful complementation of nuclease S1 analysis is the use of *E. coli* exonuclease VII. This enzyme is a progressive exonuclease that cleaves small oligonucleotides from the 5′ and 3′ ends of single-stranded DNA (38). It can therefore be used in a similar fashion to nuclease S1 or mung bean nuclease to map a transcriptional unit (39), with the exception that it will not cleave any single-stranded loops, flanked by double-stranded nucleic acid. For example, the hybrids shown in *Figure 6* would yield a different product with exonuclease VII. Fragment 1 would still be found, but fragments 2, 3, 4 and 5

72

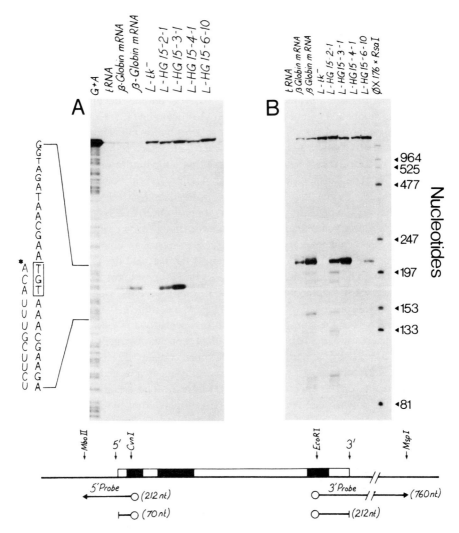

Figure 7. Nuclease S1 protection analysis of β-globin transcripts. A ³²P 5' labelled *Cvn*I-*Mbo*II fragment A or a ³²P 3' labelled *Eco*RI-*Msp*I fragment B was hybridized to mRNA from different cells. After nuclease S1 treatment, the 5' and 3' fragments were separated on 8% or 5% polyacrylamide sequence gels, respectively (37). The lanes are: G+A, the G+A cleavage product of the *Cvn*I-*Mbo*II fragment (37); tRNA as a negative control; β-globin mRNA in different quantities as a positive control; RNA from Ltk⁻ cells as a negative control; RNA from L HG cells which are different L cell clones transformed with a β-globin gene; labelled φX176 DNA restricted with *Rsa*I as a marker. The sequence of the *Cvan*I-*Mbo*II fragment is on the left. The sizes of the marker fragments are on the right.

would now be detected as larger fragments, i.e. 2/3 and 4/5 are still connected by an intron. Taken together with the nuclease S1 analysis, this would provide immediate information not only about the sizes of the exons, but also the introns. The second useful application of exonuclease VII is the detection of nuclease S1 artefacts created by partial melting of very A+T rich regions ('breathing') or repetitive sequences ('slipping') in a DNA-RNA hybrid.

73

3.8 **T7, T3 or SP6 polymerase probes**

T7, T3 and SP6 RNA polymerase are DNA dependent RNA polymerases found in cells infected with bacteriophage T7 (40), T3 (41) or SP6 (42). Each of these polymerases initiates RNA synthesis from T7, T3 or SP6 promoter sequences with very high specificity. This property can be used to synthesize single-stranded RNA from any sequence linked to such a promoter. This system was initially developed to produce large amounts of labelled precursor to study RNA processing (43). However, the RNA can also be used more effectively than DNA as a probe for DNA and RNA, because DNA-RNA and RNA-RNA hybrids in particular, are more stable than DNA-DNA hybrids. RNA-RNA hybrids have a normal melting temperature (Tm) of $94-100°C$ or $75-85°C$ in 50% formamide, whereas DNA-DNA hybrids usually have a Tm of $85-95°C$ in 50% formamide (44). The uniformly labelled RNA probes are very sensitive and allow the detection of as little as 1 pg of mRNA on Northern blots (45). This is largely due to the single-stranded nature of the probe which results in no competition with complementary sequences such as seen with double-stranded DNA probes. A practical disadvantage of this system is the fact that the DNA sequence of interest first has to be cloned next to the T7, T3 or SP6 promoter. Since it is quicker to isolate a restriction fragment than to clone it, this procedure usually means a loss of time for a single series of experiments. However, a definite gain of time is obtained when the same part of the transcriptional unit is repeatedly analysed [one cloning is, in principle (see below), quicker and cheaper than repeated fragment isolation]. There are a number of vectors commercially available which contain T7, T3 or SP6 promoters. Usually, the DNA sequences are cloned into a polylinker attached to the promoter, e.g. fragment AC of our theoretical gene (*Figure 8*). The recombinant plasmid is linearized at the downstream restriction site (C in *Figure 8*) of the inserted fragment. In the presence of labelled ribonucleotides, the polymerase initiates synthesis at the specific promoter and produces a labelled RNA transcript up to the end of the insert where the enzyme runs off the linear template. Each polymerase can transcribe the template several times and up to 10 μg of RNA can be produced from 1 μg of template DNA. The uniformly labelled RNA probe is then used in a similar fashion to the nuclease S1 DNA probes, with the exception that T1 and pancreatic ribonuclease (RNase A) are used in the protection experiment instead of nuclease S1. It should be pointed out that the synthesis is not always complete and as a consequence, the full length synthesized probe is often first purified by acrylamide gel electrophoresis to obtain optimal results. Unfortunately, this step eliminates one of the advantages (convenience) of this system. In our example, the AC probe would protect the complete first exon and half of the second exon when hybridized to mRNA. Of course, if the transcriptional unit is unknown, this method has the same advantage as S1 blotting or Northern blotting techniques when compared to end labelled probes, that is, it gives precise sizes but not the coordinates of the transcript in relation to a known position. To obtain precise coordinates, at least one other analysis with a different probe that has been restricted at a different site has to be performed. Lastly, it should be pointed out that very similar (but more cumbersome) procedures are available to synthesise uniformly labelled DNA probes from a single-stranded DNA template, using the Klenow fragment of DNA polymerase I and DNA primer (46,47).

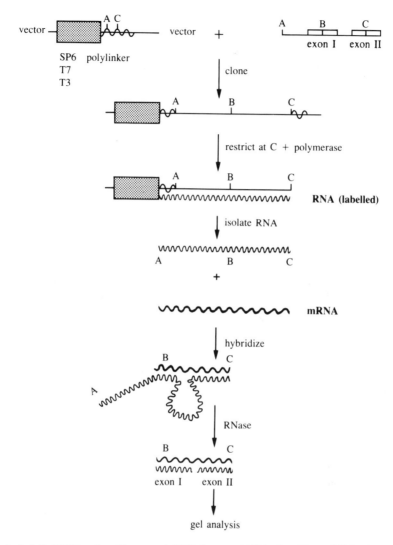

Figure 8. Labelled RNA probes. The genomic DNA fragment (AC) is cloned in a polylinker between sites A and C. The recombinant DNA is cleaved at C and transcribed into labelled RNA. After hybridization to the mRNA, the RNA-RNA hybrid is cleaved with RNase and analysed on denaturing polyacrylamide gels (37).

3.9 Primer extensions

The primer extension method is most commonly used to detect the 5′ end of splice junctions of the transcriptional unit. Moreover, just like S1 or T1 protection analysis, it can be used routinely to quantitate the levels of a particular mRNA (48). A labelled oligonucleotide or small restriction fragment is hybridized to the template mRNA and used as a primer for the synthesis of a complementary DNA by reverse transcriptase in the presence of unlabelled nucleotides. Alternatively, an unlabelled primer can be used and extended with radioactively labelled nucleotides, although the first method

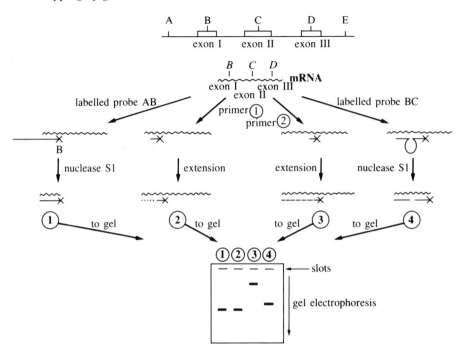

Figure 9. Primer extension analysis. The mRNA is analysed by primer extension using two labelled primers; primer 1 which is homologous to part of exon I and primer 2 which is homologous to part of exon II. Each primer is extended and the product analysed on a denaturing polyacrylamide gel (**lanes 2** and **3**). For comparison, **lanes 1** and **4** contain the products of a nuclease S1 protection experiment with labelled genomic DNA probes AB and BC respectively.

usually gives less background in the analyses. Either way, the net result is a labelled cDNA of defined length as synthesis stops at the 5′ end of the RNA (see *Figure 9*, primer 1). Measurement of the cDNA on polyacrylamide gels gives a coordinate for the 5′ end of the mRNA in relation to the known position of the primer. This method, together with a nuclease S1 protection assay is usually regarded as 'solid' evidence for the position of the 5′ end of the mRNA (e.g. 49, see *Figure 10*).

It is important to note that a number of independent but complementary techniques have to be used for definitive results to be obtained. Each method alone does not provide conclusive evidence; primer extension can give premature stops in the synthesis (strong stops), while nuclease S1 protection analysis can cleave at breathing and slippage positions (see above). Moreover, a particular nuclease S1 probe that is isolated from the first exon present in the cloned DNA might not necessarily correspond with the 5′ end of the mRNA, if another unknown exon is further upstream. Such a situation would be readily detected by the combination of procedures because the primer extension and the S1 nuclease protection analysis would give different coordinates (*Figure 9*, primer 2). Lastly, the product of a primer extension can be directly sequenced if an end-labelled primer is used. This is very convenient to locate the exact site of initiation of the mRNA and the exact intron-exon borders when the sequence is compared to the genomic DNA. Such an analysis has, for example, been used to definitely characterize the aberrant splicing event that takes place in a particular β-globin thalassaemia (50).

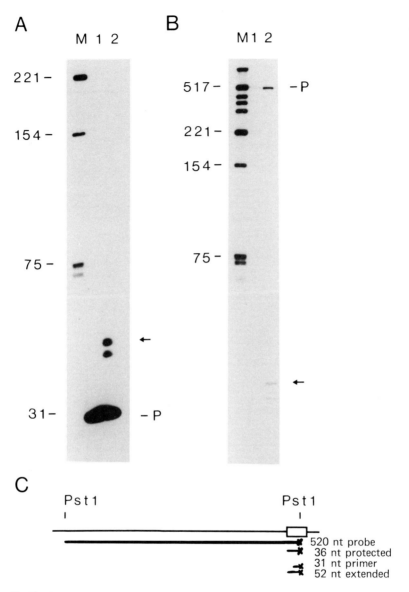

Figure 10. The 5′ end analysis of the murine Thy-1 gene. **Panel A** shows the result of a primer extension analysis using a labelled 31-nucleotide primer complementary to nucleotides (21−52) of the first exon and either 10 µg of tRNA (**lane 1**) or 25 µg of T cell RNA (**lane 2**). **Panel B** shows a nuclease S1 analysis using a labelled 520 bp Pst fragment as the probe; 36 nt of this probe are protected by T cell RNA (**lane 2**), tRNA was used as a control (**lane 1**). P is the labelled primer, the arrows indicate the extended or protected fragments. The numbers indicate the size of the marker fragments.

4. PROTOCOLS

The different protocols are the procedures we presently use in the laboratory. Some of these have evolved over several years, while others (more recent) procedures have recently been copied from others.

Table 1. Composition of solutions and buffers.

---

1. *Standard saline citrate*
   0.15 M NaCl
   0.015 M trisodium citrate

2. *10× Denhardt solution*
   0.1% bovine serum albumin
   0.1% Ficoll
   0.1% polyvinylpyrrolidone

3. *Running buffer formaldehyde for Northern blots*
   40 mM 3-N-morpholino-propane sulphonic acid (pH 7.0)
   10 mM sodium acetate
   1 mM EDTA
   2.2 M formaldehyde

4. *Sterile loading buffer*
   50% glycerol
   1 mM EDTA
   0.4% bromophenol blue
   0.4% xylene cyanol
   or 20% Ficoll
   1 mM EDTA
   0.4% orange G

5. *RSB*
   10 mM Tris-HCl (pH 7.4)
   10 mM NaCl
   5 mM $MgCl_2$

6. *Freezing buffer*
   50 mM Tris-HCl (pH 8.3)
   40% w/v glycerol
   5 mM $MgCl_2$
   0.1 mM EDTA

7. *5× 'Run-on' transcription buffer*
   25 mM Tris-HCl (pH 8.0)
   12.5 mM $MgCl_2$
   750 mM KCl
   1.25 mM ATP, GTP and CTP

8. *1× SET*
   1% SDS
   5 mM EDTA
   10 mM Tris-HCl (pH 7.4)

9. *TE*
   10 mM Tris (pH 7.5)
   1 mM EDTA

10. *Hybridization buffer for 'run-on' transcription*
    10 mM TES (pH 7.4)
    0.2% SDS
    10 mM EDTA
    300 mM NaCl
    1× Denhardt solution
    200 μg/ml *E. coli* RNA

11. *S1 buffer*
    30 mM sodium acetate (pH 4.5)
    2−4.5 mM zinc acetate
    280 mM NaCl
    This can be made and stored as 10×.

Table 1. continued.

12. *Loading buffer for nuclease S1 protection analysis*
    7 M urea
    5 mM Tris borate (pH 8.3)
    1 mM EDTA
    0.1% xylene cyanol
    0.1% bromophenol blue

13. *5× SP6 buffer*
    200 mM Tris-HCl (pH 7.5)
    30 mM $MgCl_2$
    10 mM spermidine

14. *Solution hybridization buffer for single-stranded RNA probes*
    80% formamide
    40 mM Pipes (pH 6.7)
    0.4 M NaCl
    1 mM EDTA

15. *Blot hybridization buffer for single-stranded RNA probes*
    50% formamide
    50 mM $NaPO_4$ (pH 6.5)
    5× SSC
    0.1% SDS
    5× Denhardt solution
    200 µg/ml denatured salmon sperm DNA

16. *Exonuclease VIII buffer*
    30 mM KCl
    10 mM Tris (pH 7.8)
    10 mM EDTA

4.1 Southern blots

(i)   After electrophoresis on 90 mM Tris, 90 mM boric acid, 2.5 mM EDTA (pH 8.3), soak the 0.8 cm thick agarose gels (20 × 20 cm) for 40 min in 0.2 M HCl at room temperature. This will produce depurinated sites in the DNA which can be cleaved by alkaline hydrolysis.

(ii)   Soak the gel for 40 min in 0.5 M NaOH, 1.5 M NaCl. If orange G is used as the indicator dye in the electrophoresis, it will turn red.

(iii)   Soak the gel for 40 min in 1 M Tris (pH 8.0) 3 M NaCl and transfer the gel to a blotting set-up (51) and cover by nitrocellulose filters and paper towels. Blot for 3−5 h at 4°C which is sufficient to transfer 90% or more of the nucleic acid. If the acid hydrolysis is omitted, the blotting should be much longer (overnight), because the high molecular weight DNA diffuses very slowly out of the gel. Blotting acid-treated gels overnight leads to a loss of DNA bound to the filter.

(iv)   After blotting, wash the filters (20 × 20 cm) in 2 × SSC (standard saline citrate) (see *Table 1*) and bake for 2 h at 65−80°C. Prehybridize the filter in 3 × SSC 0.1% sodium dodecylsulphate (SDS), 10 × Denhardt solution (see *Table 1*) for 2 h at 65°C. Hybridize in 5−20 ml of 3 × SSC 10 × Denhardts, 0.1% SDS, 10% dextran sulphate and denatured labelled probe for 6−12 h at 65°C. Depending on the probes, various competitors can be added to the hybridization, in addition to 50 µg/ml denatured salmon sperm DNA.

Table 2. Recipe for ^{35}S-labelled RNA probes.

		Final conc.
5 × SP6 buffer[a]	4 µl	1×
BSA 5 mg/ml	0.4 µl	100 µg/ml
Triton X-100 5%	0.5 µl	0.1%
rNTP (C+A+G 10 mM each)	1 µl	0.5 mM
DTT 0.5 M	0.5 µl	12 mM
SP6 polymerase (dil 1:10)	0.5 µl (=1.25 U)	
RNAsin (inhibitor, 1 U/µl)	0.5 µl	25 U/ml
[^{32}P]- or [^{35}S]UTP	10 µl	~4 µM
1.2 µg linearized DNA (2 kb insert)		~60 µg/ml
Add H$_2$O to a final volume of 20 µl		

[a]See *Table 1* for composition of 5× SP6 buffer

(v)　Wash the filters twice for 20 min in 3 × SSC, 0.1% SDS at 65°C, twice in 0.3 × SSC, 0.1% SDS at 65°C and for stringent hybridizations, conditions are 0.1 × SSC, 0.1% SDS at 65°C. After a final wash in 2 × SSC at room temperature for 2 min dry the filters and expose them to X-ray film using cassettes and intensifying screens.

Note: There are several non-nitrocellulose filters on the market, which are blotted and hybridized as specified by the manufacturers. These filters are stronger, can be re-used more often and at least some bind very low molecular weight fragments much more efficiently. Unfortunately, they are more expensive.

4.2 Northern blots

(i)　Dissolve the RNA (1−20 µg) in 10−20 µl of running buffer formaldehyde (see *Table 1*) and incubate at 55°C for 15 min. Add 2−5 µl of sterile loading buffer (see *Table 1*).

(ii)　Melt agarose (1−2% final concentration), cool to 60°C, add 5× running buffer and formaldehyde.

(iii)　After electrophoresis the marker lanes can be cut off, stained in 0.5 µg/ml ethidium bromide and visualized on a u.v. transilluminator (51). Rinse the remainder of the gel in water for 5 min, then soak it for 40 min in 50 mM NaOH, 10 mM NaCl to partially hydrolyse the RNA which improves the transfer of high molecular weight material. Neutralize the gel in 1.0 M Tris (pH 7.0), 1.5 M NaCl, for 40 min and transfer as Southern gels.

4.3 'Run-on' transcription (52)

(i)　Wash tissue culture cells with ice cold phosphate-buffered saline (PBS) and trypsinize from the plates. Wash complete tissues in PBS and homogenize with the aid of a Dounce homogenizer. All further steps are at 0°C unless stated otherwise.

(ii)　Pellet the cells at 500 *g* for 5 min, wash them once in RSB (see *Table 1*) and repellet at 500 *g* for 5 min.

(iii)   Resuspend the cells in RSB plus 0.5% NP-40 and release the nuclei by *gentle* agitation in a Dounce homogenizer.

(iv)   Pellet the nuclei at 500 *g* for 5 min and resuspend them in 100 μl of freezing buffer (see *Table 1*) at a concentration of $10^7 - 10^8$ nuclei/100 μl and freeze at $-70°C$.

(v)   Add 210 μl of thawed nuclei to 60 μl of 5× 'run-on' buffer (see *Table 1*) per reaction. Add 30 μl of α-[^{32}P]UTP (3200 Ci/mM) and incubate the suspension at 30°C for 30 min.

(vi)   Add 15 μl of 5 μg/m DNase I in 10 mM $CaCl_2$ and incubate at 30°C for 5 min. Stop the reaction by the addition of 5 × SET to a final concentration of 1 × SET (see *Table 1*).

(vii)   Add proteinase K (20 mg/ml) to a final concentration of 200 μg/ml and incubate for 45 min at 37°C.

(viii)   Extract the RNA with an equal volume of phenol/chloroform (1:1) and centrifuge. Re-extract the interphase with 100 μl of 1 × SET and re-centrifuge. Make the combined aqueous phases 2.3 M NH_4OAc (10 M stock) and add an equal volume of isopropanol. After 15 min at $-70°C$ pellet the nuclei acid in a microfuge for 10 min.

(ix)   Dissolve the pellet in 100 μl of TE (see *Table 1*). Centrifuge the sample or run the sample over a G-50 column. Make the eluate 0.2 M NaOH and keep it on ice for 10 min. Add Hepes to a final concentration of 0.24 M for neutralization and precipitate the nucleic acid by the addition of 2.5 volumes of ethanol, stored at $-20°C$. Pellet the nucleic acid in a microfuge (10 min). Resuspend the pelleted labelled RNA in $2-5$ ml of hybridization buffer (see *Table 1*).

(x)   Bind the restriction fragments (0.5-5 μg) to the nitrocellulose filters with the aid of a Schleicher and Schull Slot Blot apparatus as suggested by the manufacturers.

(xi)   Pre-hybridize the filters at 65°C in hybridization buffer and transfer to the hybridization solution containing the [^{32}P]RNA. Hybridize for 36 h at 65°C. Wash the filters twice for 15 min in 2 × SSC, 0.1% SDS at room temperature and once at 60°C in 0.1 × SSC, 0.1% SDS for 30 min.

(xii)   Expose the filters to Kodak XAR film in cassettes with intensifying screens at $-70°C$. Quantitate the 'slots' by scanning or counting in a scintillation counter. Correct the final quantities for the length of the DNA fragment and (if known) the T content (the label was only in UTP).

4.4 Nuclease S1 protection analysis

(i)   Label 100 ng of probe by kinasing or 'filling in', which is enough for 20 lanes approximately. Otherwise, go directly to step (ii).

(ii)   Dissolve the probe in hybridization buffer [80% formamide (recrystallized or at least deionized), 0.04 M Pipes (pH 6.4), 1 mM EDTA, 0.4 M NaCl].

(iii)   Precipitate the RNA (5-50 μg of RNA per lane depending on how abundant the mRNA is) in ethanol (2.5 vol), spin and dissolve the pellet in $10-30$ μl of hybridization buffer with the probe.

(iv)   Place at 90°C for 5 min to denature the RNA and DNA probe and transfer immediately into a 52°C water-bath and hybridize for a minimum of 6 h to overnight. Have the two waterbaths next to each other. We do the hybridization in Eppendorf tubes and keep them sealed by clamping the lids between the holding rack and a solid cover (plastic or metal). Keep the surface of the water in the two baths to the neck of the tubes.

(v)   While the tubes are still in the waterbath, just open the lids; do not lift out until you add 10 volumes of S1 buffer (see *Table 1*) containing 30 units of S1 nuclease (Boehringer). Then vortex and put in ice until all the tubes are done.

(vi)   Transfer into a 20°C waterbath for 2 h (certain probes need different temperatures, 20−40°C), extract with phenol:chloroform and ethanol precipitate. Dissolve the pellet in 5 μl loading buffer (see *Table 1*).

(vii)   Run on a sequence gel (37) or agarose gels if blotting is required.

4.5 Single-stranded RNA probes

Transcription (D.Ish-Horowitz, personal communication) − hybridization (53). The recipe for ^{35}S-probe is given in *Table 2*.

(i)   Incubate the ^{35}S-probe mixture for ≥ 1 h at 30°C (up to 4 h).

(ii)   Make reaction 1 × MS [10 mM Tris (pH 7.5), 10 mM MgCl$_2$, 50 mM NaCl], add 1/10 vol. RNase-free DNase (53) (20−50 μg/ml) and incubate at 37°C for 30 min.

(iii)   Add EDTA to 20 mM, SDS to 0.2%, 5 μg tRNA carrier and spin through Biogel P-60 or Sephadex G-50 column.

(iv)   Separate the full length transcript on polyacrylamide gels (37) if the final analysis has a high background due to incomplete RNA synthesis or incomplete digestion of the DNA template.

Notes: The K_m for UTP is high, UTP concentration must be >2 μM or there will be substantial premature termination, >10 μM is better. If necessary, dilute the label with cold triphosphate. CTP has a lower K_m and is better for making full length probes. The lower incubation temperature (30°C) and 0.1% Triton favours longer transcripts. Salt in the reaction promotes premature termination and should be avoided. Also, NH$_4$$^+$ is a potent inhibitor of the SP6 polymerase. For hotter probes, use T7 polymerase. T7 polymerase also has a lower K_m for UTP so it is easier to use with labelled UTP.
    The above recipe works for T7 with the following modifications:

    (i)   Use about four units of T7 polymerase per reaction.
    (ii)   Avoid labelled GTP, this has a high K_m.

(v)   Dissolve the test RNA (5−40 μg) and the labelled probe RNA in 30 μl of solution hybridization buffer (see *Table 1*). Denature at 85°C for 5 min and incubate (>8 h) at 45°C. Different temperatures are optimal depending on the G+C content of the hybrid.

(vi)   Add 300 μl of 0.3 M NaCl, 10 mM Tris-HCl (pH 7.5), 5 mM EDTA, RNase A (40 μg/ml) and RNase T1 (2 μg/ml) and incubate for 1 h at 30°C. Again different temperatures might be used to obtain the best signal to background ratio.

(vii)   Stop the RNase digestion by the addtiion of 20 μl 10% SDS and 50 μg of proteinase K. Incubate for 15 min at 37°C. Extract with phenol/chloroform and precipitate the labelled RNA hybrids with 5 μg tRNA in 2 × volumes of ethanol. Spin and dissolve the pellet in S1 loading buffer and run on 8 M urea-polyacrylamide gels (37).

(viii)   If the probes are required for Southern or Northern blots, proceed from step (iii) to dissolving the probe in blot hybridization buffer and hybridize at 55 − 60°C. Wash as for Southern blotting protocol.

4.6 Exonuclease VII digestion

(i)   The hybridizations are carried out exactly as described for the nuclease S1 protocols; proceed as from Section 4.4 step (iv).

(ii)   Add 500 μl of exonuclease VII buffer (see *Table 1*) with 4 U/ml exonuclease VII. Incubate for 2 h at 37°C. Extract with phenol/chloroform, ethanol precipitate and proceed exactly as described for the nuclease S1 protocol step (vi) and (vii).

4.7 Primer extensions

(i)   After labelling, isolate the synthetic primer or the primer restriction fragment from a preparative agarose gel or polyacrylamide gel (depending on its size) and ethanol precipitate.

(ii)   Dissolve 10 − 30 μg of total RNA and about 0.2 pmol of the labelled primer in 10 μl of 400 mM NaCl, 10 mM Pipes (pH 6.4). Seal the mixture in a glass capilary, denature at 90°C for 2 min and hybridize overnight at 30°C.

Note: The amounts of RNA and primer depend on the relative abundance in the total RNA population. The hybridization temperature depends on the length of the primer, the conditions described above are for a 30-mer.

(iii)   Primer extension is started by delivering the hybridization mixture into the extension mixture containing 50 mM Tris-HCl (pH 8.2), 10 mM DTT, 6 mM $MgCl_2$, 0.5 mM of each dNTP, 2.5 μg actinomycin D and 10 units of reverse transcriptase. Incubate the reaction at 41°C for 1 h. Stop the reaction by the addition of 0.1% SDS, 10 mM EDTA (final concentrations) and extract the products with phenol/chloroform and precipitate with ethanol.

(iv)   Run the extension products, with or without sequencing, on denaturing polyacrylamide gels (37).

5. REFERENCES

1.   Glover,D.M. (1985) *DNA Cloning − A Practical Approach*, Vol. **1**, published by IRL Press, Oxford.
2.   Karn,J. (1983) *Techniques in the Life Sciences. Nucleic Acid Biochemistry, B501*, Vol. B5, published by Elsevier Scientific Publishers Ireland Ltd.
3.   Grosveld,F.G. and Dahl,H.H.M .(1983) *Techniques in the Life Sciences. Nucleic Acid Biochemistry, B502*, Vol. **B5**, published by Elsevier Scientific Publishers Ireland Ltd.
4.   Chang,A., Nurnberg,J., Kaufman,R., Ehrlich,H., Schimke,R. and Cohen,S. (1978) *Nature*, **275**, 617.
5.   Nagata,S., Taira,H., Hall,A., Johnsrud,L., Streuli,M., Escodi,J., Boll,W., Canell,K. and Weissmann,C. (1980) *Nature*, **284**, 316.
6.   Wallace,M.B., Johnson,M.J., Hirose,T., Miyake,T., Kawashima,E.K. and Itakura,K. (1982) *Nucleic Acids Res.*, **9**, 879.
7.   Kuhn,L.C., McClelland,A. and Ruddle,F.H. (1984) *Cell*, **37**, 95.
8.   Littman,D.R., Thomas,Y., Madon,P.J., Chess,L. and Axel,R. (1985) *Cell*, **40**, 237.
9.   Kavathas,P., Sukhatine,V.P., Herzenberg,C.A. and Parnes,J.R. (1984) *Proc. Natl. Acad. Sci. USA*, **81**, 7688.

10. Anderson,D.J. and Axel,R. (1985) *Cell*, **42**, 649.
11. Sharp,P.A. (1985) *Cell*, **42**, 397.
12. Birnstiel,M.L., Busslinger,M. and Strub,K. (1985) *Cell*, **41**, 349.
13. Boseley,P.G. (1983) *Techniques in the Life Sciences. Nucleic Acid Biochemistry*, Vol. **B5**, published by Elsevier Scientific Publishers Ireland Ltd.
14. Southern,E.M. (1975) *J. Mol. Biol.*, **98**, 503.
15. Jeffreys,A.J. and Flavell,R.A. (1977) *Cell*, **12**, 1097.
16. Alwine,J.C., Kemp,D.J. and Stark,G.R. (1977) *Proc. Natl. Acad. Sci. USA*, **74**, 5350.
17. Chambon,P., Benoist,C., Breathnach,R., Cochet,M., Cannon,F., Gerlinger,P., Knist,A., LeMeur,M., LePennec,J.P., Mandel,J.L., O'Hare,K. and Perrin,F. (1979) in *From Gene to Protein. Information transfer in normal and abnormal cells.* Russell,R., Brew,K., Faber,H. and Schultz,J. (eds.), Academic Press, New York, Vol. **16**, p. 55.
18. Zeitlin,S. and Efstratiadis,A. (1984) *Cell*, **39**, 589.
19. Hofer,E. and Darnell,J.E. (1981) *Cell*, **23**, 585.
20. Weber,J., Jelinek,W. and Darnell,J.E. (1977) *Cell*, **10**, 611.
21. Blanchard,J.M., Weber,J., Jelinek,W. and Darnell,J.E. (1979) *Proc. Natl. Acad. Sci. USA*, **75**, 5344.
22. Salditt-Georgief,M. and Darnell,J.E. (1983) *Proc. Natl. Acad. Sci. USA*, **80**, 4694 and **81**, 2274.
23. LeMuer,M.A., Galliot,B. and Gerlinger,P. (1984) *EMBO J.*, **3**, 2779.
24. White,R.L. and Hogness,D.S. (1977) *Cell*, **10**, 177.
25. Birnstiel,M.L., Sells,B.H. and Purdom,T. (1972) *J. Mol. Biol.*, **63**, 21.
26. Casey,J. and Davidson,N. (1977) *Nucleic Acids Res.*, **4**, 1539.
27. Tilghman,S.M., Tiemeier,D.C., Seidman,J.G., Peterlin,B.M., Sullivan,M., Maizel,J.V. and Leder,P. (1978) *Proc. Natl. Acad. Sci. USA*, **75**, 725.
28. Berk,A.J. and Sharp,P.A. (1977) *Cell*, **12**, 721.
29. Vogt,V.M. (1973) *Eur. J. Biochem.*, **33**, 192.
30. Laskowski,M. (1980) in *Methods in Enzymology*, Vol. **65**, Grossman,L. and Moldave,K. (eds), Academic Press, New York, p. 263.
31. Grosveld,G.C., Koster,A. and Flavell,R.A. (1981) *Cell*, **23**, 573.
32. Weaver,R.F. and Weissmann,C. (1979) *Nucleic Acids Res.*, **6**, 1175.
33. Richardson,C.C. (1971) *Proc. Natl. Acad. Sci. USA*, **72**, 815.
34. Jacobson,H., Klenow,H., Overgaard-Hansen,K. (1974) *Eur. J. Biochem.*, **45**, 623.
35. Sanger,F. and Coulson,A.R. (1975) *J. Mol. Biol.*, **94**, 441.
36. Verma,I.M. (1977) *Biochem. Biophys. Acta*, **473**, 1.
37. Maxam,A.M. and Gilbert,W. (1980) in *Methods in Enzymology*, Vol. **65**, Grossman,L. and Moldave,K. (eds), Academic Press, New York, p. 499.
38. Chase,J.W. and Richardson,C.C. (1964) *J. Biol. Chem.*, **249**, 4545.
39. Berk,A.J. and Sharp,P.A. (1978) *Cell*, **14**, 695.
40. Chamberlain,M., McGrath,J. and Waskell,L. (1979) *Nature*, **288**, 227.
41. Chamberlain,M., McGrath,J. and Waskell,L. (1970) *Nature*, **228**, 227.
42. Butler,E.T. and Chamberlain,M.J. (1982) *J. Biol. Chem.*, **257**, 5772.
43. Green,M.R., Maniatis,T. and Melton,D.A. (1983) *Cell*, **32**, 681.
44. Cox,K.H,. deLeon,D.V., Augerer,C.M. and Augerer,R.C. (1984) *Dev. Biol.*, **101**, 485.
45. Zinn,K., Maio,D. and Maniatis,T. (1983) *Cell*, **34**, 865.
46. Rica,G.A., Taylor,J.M. and Kalinyak,J.E. (1982) *Proc. Natl. Acad. Sci. USA*, **79**, 724.
47. Antoniou,M., Guzman,K., Chakraborty,S. and Banerjee,M.R. (1985) *J. Biophys. Biochem. Methods*, **11**, 208.
48. McKnight,S.L., Garis,E.R. and Kingsbury,R. (1981) *Cell*, **25**, 385.
49. Giguere,V., Ishobe,K.-I. and Grosveld,F.G. (1985) *EMBO J.*, **4**, 2017.
50. Busslinger,M., Moschonas,N. and Flavell,R.A. (1981) *Cell*, **27**, 289.
51. Maniatis,T., Fritsch,E.F. and Sambrook,J. (1982) *Molecular Cloning. A Laboratory Manual*, published by Cold Spring Harbor Laboratory Press, NY.
52. Linial,M., Ginderson,N. and Groudine,M. (1985) *Science*, **230**, 1126.
53. Melton,D.A., Krieg,P.A., Rebagliati,M.R., Maniatis,T., Zinn,Z. and Green,M.R. (1984) *Nucleic Acids Res.*, **12**, 7035.
54. Maxwell,I.H., Maxwell,E. and Mahn,W.E. (1977) *Nucleic Acids Res.*, **4**, 241.

CHAPTER 6

In situ hybridization

VERONICA J. BUCKLE and IAN W. CRAIG

1. INTRODUCTION

A variety of strategies is available for the localization of cloned genes and random DNA sequences within the human genome. One approach involves hybridization to a panel of DNA obtained from somatic cell hybrids with different human chromosomes present. For regional localization within a particular chromosome, sequences can be hybridized to the DNA from cell lines carrying deletions of that chromosome, and thereby mapped within or outside the deletion. A panel of somatic cell hybrids with various rearrangements of a particular chromosome can also be used in this way. The smallest region of overlap which gives a positive hybridization signal can then be determined. The preceding strategies require detailed cytogenetic characterizations of the cell lines being used, and for regional assignments must rely on the accuracy and precision with which the break points of all these structural abnormalities have been defined. *In situ* hybridization provides a direct approach to regional mapping. Nucleic acid sequences can be directly hybridized *in situ* to their complementary DNA within fixed chromosome preparations on glass slides. After autoradiography, a significant excess of silver grains may be scored within one region of a particular chromosome. This procedure will also indicate whether any other sites of hybridization are present within the genome.

The hybridization of RNA to the DNA of a cytological preparation was first described by Gall and Pardue in 1969 (1), who demonstrated spatial localization in the hybridization of ribosomal RNA to *Xenopus* oocytes, detected by tritium autoradiography. The general principles of the technique they developed remain the basis of contemporary studies. The most important are the removal of basic proteins from the cytological preparation by acid-fixation, the denaturation of chromosomal DNA whilst retaining cytological integrity, hybridization under conditions enabling specific pairing and autoradiography with a liquid emulsion.

Since the early 1970s this procedure has been used to localize sequences repeated many times within the human genome, with easily purified RNA or DNA. A major obstacle to the localization of other specific gene sequences was the lack of probes of sufficient purity. The advent of DNA recombinant technology meant that DNA sequences could be prepared free of other hybridizing contaminants, which resulted in a major improvement in the resolution of the signal obtained. This, together with improvements in the efficiency of hybridization and in the quality of chromosome banding, have made the technique of *in situ* hybridization sufficiently sensitive to permit the localization of single copy sequence DNA. It has therefore become an important complement to the use of deletion cell lines, somatic cell hybrids and linkage analysis, in the mapping of human sequences.

2. THEORETICAL BASIS OF THE TECHNIQUE

The hybridization *in situ* of single-stranded DNA, or RNA, to chromosome preparations requires several sequential procedures. These stages will be considered separately and the variable practical parameters will be discussed. Reference 2 provides a review of the behaviour of nucleic acids in solution and the application of elements of that behaviour to the method of *in situ* hybridization.

2.1 Preparation of target material

An aceto-methanol fixative will remove basic proteins which may otherwise interfere with hybridization. An alternative fixative must be chosen with care because of possible effects on the autoradiographic emulsion by chemography or latent image fading (3). Through the many stages of the technique the cytological material can become detached from the glass slide and lost. A pre-treatment of the glass with poly-lysine or gelatin and chrome-alum can control this and may assist in the adhesion of the emulsion, but will interfere with good chromosome spreading and is unnecessary, provided that care is exercised throughout the procedure.

Native RNA within the chromosome preparations can compete for binding sites with the radioactive input and labelled cDNA or cRNA can form duplexes with cytoplasmic RNA. Native RNA must therefore be removed prior to hybridization to avoid both low hybridization efficiency and high background signal.

DNA molecules can be denatured to their constituent single strands by heat and by exposure to strong acid or alkaline conditions. A high $G+C$ content in the DNA confers a higher thermal stability as does increasing salt concentration. Chaotropic agents such as formamide reduce the thermal stability of DNA. Several methods have been used to denature the DNA of cytological preparations: sodium hydroxide (1), hydrochloric acid (4), heat in the presence of formamide (5). The use of formamide to lower the thermal stability of DNA allows preservation of chromosome morphology with suitable hybridization efficiency and this has been the method of choice in the authors' laboratory.

2.2 Radioactive isotopes

In order to be suitable for *in situ* hybridization, a radioactive isotope must have a high specific activity and give good resolution. The distance an emitted particle will travel through the photographic emulsion depends on the initial particle energy (3):

Initial energy (keV)	Track length (Ilford G5 emulsion) (μm)
10	1
20	2.9
30	6
40	10

The merits of three isotopes, ^3H, ^{125}I and ^{35}S will be considered here.

2.2.1 ^3H

Tritium has a specific activity of $50-85$ Ci/mmol with a half-life of 12.3 years. It emits beta particles with a maximum particle energy of 18 keV and an average energy of 9−12 keV. The short range that these weak beta particles are able to travel through photographic emulsion (1 μm) permits precise localization of the source. A disadvantage of using a tritiated probe is the long exposure time required for detection of unique sequences.

2.2.2 ^{125}I

The principle advantage of ^{125}I is its high specific activity (1500 Ci/mmol) due to a relatively short half-life of 60 days. Consequently, probe DNA can be labelled to a high specific activity by the introduction of limited quantities of ^{125}I atoms. ^{125}I decays by internal conversion and a variety of particles are emitted with a wide range of energies:

Particle energy (keV)	2.77	3.6	22.5	31	34.3
% of electrons emitted	28	49	14	7	1

Seventy seven percent of electrons emitted have a particle energy of less than 4 keV. Thus, at the expense of a higher background, good resolution is obtainable with this isotope.

2.2.3 ^{35}S

This has a half-life of 87.2 days, and emits beta particles with a high energy (50 keV average). Although high specific activities are obtainable with ^{35}S-labelled probes, such high initial energies make the isotope unsuitable for work requiring high resolution.

2.3 Nucleic acid reassociation

The optimal DNA/DNA reassociation temperature (*Tr*) occurs some 25°C below the 'melting point' (*Tm*) of the corresponding native duplex (6), whilst the *Tr* for RNA/DNA hybrids occurs closer to the *Tm* of that hybrid. Stringent conditions of lower salt concentration and higher temperature favour accurate base pairing. The presence of formamide will lower the *Tr* and so help maintain chromosome morphology. The rate of reassociation is concentration dependent, and therefore is higher for simple (repetitive) sequences than for more complex sequences. Dextran sulphate has been shown to increase the rate of reassociation with DNA (7) and carrier salmon sperm DNA may be included to reduce non-specific binding of labelled probe.

Cloned genomic DNA or complementary DNA is the normal choice of probe in hybridization reactions, and the whole vector with insert is used in order to enhance the signal at the site of hybridization. Incorporation of radiolabel by nick-translation results in randomly cleaved molecules of variable length. The presence of radiolabelled sequences in the hybridization mixture can lead to the formation of extensive DNA networks, either in solution or at the chromosomal site being probed (8). The production of RNA transcript labelled to high specific activity employing the SP6 vector system provides a controlled procedure for obtaining single-stranded probes but has yet to be fully evaluated in this context.

2.4 Post-hybridization treatment

RNA/DNA hybrids are resistant to RNase so, where RNA has been used as a probe, a mild RNase treatment will remove non-base-paired RNA. After DNA/DNA annealing there is no enzymatic means of removing non-base-paired DNA and this must therefore be achieved by extensive washing in $2-0.1 \times$ SSC. Manipulation of salt concentration and temperature can remove less well-matched hybrids as well as controlling non-specific background.

2.5 **Autoradiographic emulsion**

After washing, the slides are dipped in a liquid emulsion and left to expose at 4°C. Dipping emulsion is composed of a matrix of gelatin in which crystals of silver bromide are embedded. The crystal size varies in different emulsions between 0.07 and 0.4 μm. Silver bromide forms a regular crystal lattice and each crystal will have some faults. Orbital electrons in the crystals may acquire enough energy from particles emitted from the labelled site of hybridization to leave their orbits. Displaced electrons can interact with faults in the crystals to deposit metallic silver (the latent image). Clearly the larger the crystal, the longer the particle track will be and the more silver will be deposited. Similarly, the slower the emitted particle, the more interactions with orbital electrons will take place and the more silver will be deposited at that site. Conversely the smaller the crystal size or the more energetic the particle, the less silver will be deposited. Resolution of signal in the emulsion can be optimized by selection of small crystal size, particles with a low initial energy, which will produce less scatter of signal, and a thin emulsion layer. The crystal size of Ilford L4 emulsion is 0.14 μm and of Kodak NTB-2 is 0.26 μm. These are the two most suitable emulsions for detecting tritiated or iodinated hybridization complexes.

Latent image fading, where the silver atom rejoins the crystal lattice, can occur during exposure in the presence of moisture or oxidizing agents.

Development of the emulsion reduces silver bromide to metallic silver. Reduction occurs faster where metallic silver is already present, therefore careful control of development is required to obtain the most informative latent image to background ratio. Development time is affected by temperature, concentration and agitation of the developer solution.

2.6 **Chromosome banding**

Banding procedures are used in conjunction with the technique of *in situ* hybridization to permit unambiguous assignments to specific chromosomes. Improving techniques admit the potential for assigning sequences to specific chromosomal bands.

Evans *et al.* (9) and Gosden *et al.* (4) used Q banding by quinacrine dihydrochloride. They photographed selected cells, performed the hybridization then relocated the same cells for analysis of grain distribution. They compared Q-banded and post-hybridization photographs of each chromosome in order to plot the distribution of silver grains. This approach has some advantage in terms of objectivity, but is extremely time-consuming and not sufficiently accurate to allow location of silver grains to specific bands. Furthermore, such pre-treatment to the chromosome preparations may affect the subsequent efficiency of hybridization. A method of banding after hybridization was described by Chandler and Yunis (5) using Wrights stain. They stained, de-stained and re-stained through the emulsion several times to obtain a combination of G and C banding. Published banded photographs from this group are of a high quality but many other workers have been unable to obtain banding of a similar consistent quality by this method. Lawrie and Gosden (10) reported a method for Q banding, after hybridization and before the emulsion dip, which allowed silver grains to be observed directly on Q-banded chromosomes. The drawback to this approach is that chromosomal fluorescence fades with direct exposure to u.v. light, whilst repeated reference to a cell under the microscope rather than by photograph is required for a detailed analysis of silver grain distribution.

Zabel *et al.* (11) incorporated the method of replication banding (12) into their *in situ* hybridization procedure. Bromodeoxyuridine (BUdR) is added to a cell culture in such a concentration that it blocks synthesis in the middle of S-phase and the cells become synchronized at this point. Prior to the block in synthesis, BUdR will have been incorporated into early replicating regions of the chromosomes. After release of the block, and continued culture in thymidine-enriched medium, the synchronized population of cells can be harvested when they reach mitosis without the use of colcemid. Subsequent Hoechst−u.v.−Giemsa staining results in replication-banded chromosomes where BUdR-incorporated regions (early replicating) appear as pale bands and thymidine-incorporated regions (late replicating) stain darkly. Replication banding corresponds closely to G banding (13) although the two patterns may not be identical. This banding technique is particularly useful in conjunction with *in situ* hybridization since only Hoechst and Giemsa stains are required to penetrate the emulsion.

An alternative approach to good regional assignment by *in situ* hybridization is the use of meiotic rather than mitotic chromosome preparations. Jhanwar *et al.* (14) observed a close correspondence of the chromomere maps of mid-pachytene spermatocytes with the 850-stage banding pattern (15) of somatic chromosomes, and the group have since published several '*in situ*' assignments using meiotic preparations (16−18). Good resolution is possible, no banding procedures are required and the authors suggest a possible enhancement of signal due to homologous pairing of the bivalents. However, material may not be readily available and this approach is not applicable to studies involving the sex chromosomes since their morphology in pachytene is obscured in the sex vesicle.

2.7 Setting up the technique in the laboratory

If the technique has not been previously attempted, a stepwise approach is recommended before working with single copy sequences of unknown location. Initial experiments are best performed using a highly repetitive sequence as probe. This will ensure a detectable signal whilst any major problems with the technique are resolved. Once a reliable signal is obtained with such a probe, the use of a single copy sequence of known chromosomal assignment is a good test of the accuracy and sensitivity of the technique. It should then be possible to localize sequences of unknown chromosomal origin with some confidence.

3. PROTOCOL

3.1 Preparation of slides and coverslips

Slides and coverslips should be cleaned before use. Soak in strong detergent (e.g. Lipsol, Decon) overnight, then rinse in distilled water and soak in a weak HCl solution for 1−2 h. Rinse thoroughly in distilled water, soak in ethanol and air dry.

3.2 **Preparation of chromosomes**

This technique gives replication G banding and avoids the problems associated with the alternative techniques of pre-banding and photographing spreads, or post-banding through a layer of emulsion.

(i)   To prepare phytohaemagglutinin (PHA)-stimulated lymphocytes, add 0.4 ml of whole blood to each culture bottle containing 5 ml of McCoy's medium (see *Table 1*), with PHA, and culture for 72 h at 37°C. Where lymphoblastoid cell lines are used, grow until a healthy dividing population is obtained, with around 5×10^6 cells per 10 ml of culture medium. See Section 6 for details of culture media.

(ii) Add BUdR to a concentration of 200 μg/ml of medium and incubate the culture for $16-17$ h. During this time the cell cycle becomes blocked in the middle of S-phase and the cells are synchronized at that point.

(iii) Wash the cells twice by centrifuging at 1000 r.p.m. for 5 min and resuspend in fresh medium, in order to remove all trace of the BUdR and thereby release the block in the cell cycle.

(iv) Resuspend in fresh medium containing 10^{-5} M thymidine and continue to culture for a further $6-7$ h. Colcemid is unnecessary as the cell population is now synchronized.

(v)   Centrifuge the cells as before, discard the supernatant and resuspend in a hypotonic solution of 0.56% KCl, previously warmed to 37°C, and leave at that temperature for 10 min.

(vi) Centrifuge, discard the supernatant and resuspend the cells in a freshly prepared fixative of three parts Analar methanol to one part glacial acetic acid. Add the fixative a drop at a time, up to 7 ml, mixing thoroughly. Leave for 20 min at 4°C, then wash repeatedly with fresh fixative until the cell suspension is clean.

(vii) Place a drop of cell suspension on each glass slide and allow to air dry. Check the quality of preparation on a test slide under phase contrast. Slides can be used the day after they are made. They will keep for approximately 5 weeks, or longer if stored in a sealed container with desiccant at -40°C.

Note. From the time of addition of BUdR until after hybridization, cells and slides should be protected from direct light to avoid nicking of the BUdR-incorporated DNA. Work under safelight in a darkroom if possible, and wrap the slides in a black plastic bag when transferring from room to room.

(viii) Stain a test slide to ensure that the BUdR has been incorporated correctly. Immerse in a solution of Hoechst 33258 (Sigma; B2883) diluted 2 μg/ml in 2 × SSC (see *Table 1*) for 30 min. Rinse in 2 × SSC, place the slide flat in a Petri dish and cover completely with 2 × SSC. Place the Petri dish 20 cm from a long-wave u.v. light source (Sylvania; Blacklite-blue) for 1 h. Stain the slide for 3 min in 10% Giemsa (BDH; 35086) diluted in pH 6.8 phosphate buffer. Rinse in the same buffer and air dry.

3.3 **Treatment of slides prior to hybridization**

Throughout the procedure slides should be handled with care and moved gently from

Table 1. Composition of media and solutions.

McCoy's 5A medium

To 100 ml of medium (Flow; 12-552-49) add:
2 ml	phytohaemagglutinin (Gibco; 061-0576C)
2000 units	heparin (BDH; 28470)
20 ml	foetal calf serum
200 mM	L-glutamine (Imperial Laboratories; 4-701-07)
10 000 units	penicillin
10 mg	streptomycin.

RPMI medium

To 100 ml of medium (Imperial Laboratories; 2-540-14) add:
10 ml	foetal calf serum
200 mM	L-glutamine
10 000 units	penicillin
10 mg	streptomycin.

Hybridization fluid

For 1 ml:
500 μl	formamide AR
100 μl	50 × Denhardt's solution
400 μl	25% dextran sulphate in 12.5 × SSPE
20 μl	10 mg/ml stock solution of salmon sperm DNA.

Denhardt's solution (50 ×)

Ficoll 400	0.1 g
Polyvinylpyrrolidine 360	0.1 g
Bovine serum albumin	0.1 g
Dilute to 10 ml with distilled water.	

SSPE (12.5 ×)

NaCl	1.3 g
NaH_2PO_4	0.2 g
EDTA	0.046 g
Dilute to 10 ml with distilled water	

SSC (20 ×)

Sodium chloride	175 g
Tri-sodium citrate	88 g
Dilute to 1 litre with distilled water.	

D19 developer

Sodium sulphite, anhydrous	90 g
Sodium carbonate, anhydrous	45 g
Quinol	8 g
Potassium bromide	5 g
Metol	2 g
Dilute to 1 litre with distilled water.	

one solution to another, in a glass slide rack wherever possible, in order to prevent loss of material from the surface of the slide.

(i)   Prepare a stock solution of RNase (Sigma; R5500) for use by boiling for 10 min to remove any contaminating DNase, cool slowly to room temperature and store frozen until required. Use at a concentration of 100 μg/ml in 2 × SSC. Place 150 μl of this solution on each slide under a coverslip, and incubate in a moist chamber at 37°C for 1 h. A plastic sandwich box with a sheet of filter paper, moistened with 2 × SSC, can be used for this purpose.

(ii)   Dip the slides in 2 × SSC to allow the coverslips to float off, wash in three changes of 2 × SSC, dehydrate through an alcohol series (30 sec in each of 10, 50, 75, 95 and 100% ethanol) and air dry.

(iii)   Denature the chromosomal DNA by incubating the slides in 70% formamide/ 0.1 mM EDTA in 2 × SSC, for 4 min at 65°C. Then treat the slides as before: wash, dehydrate through an alcohol series and air dry. They can be stored in a desiccator for a short time if necessary.

3.4 Hybridization

The quantities of DNA, hybridization solution, etc. given in this part of the method are sufficient to treat 10 slides, which is the number considered necessary to encompass variations in the stringency of washing and in the length of exposure when attempting a *de novo* assignment of a DNA sequence.

(i)   Label 100 ng of probe DNA by nick-translation with either [^{3}H]dCTP (Amersham; TRK625) or [^{125}I]dCTP (Amersham; IM5103) using a standard nick-translation kit (Amersham; N5000) according to the manufacturer's instructions. Incorporation of [^{125}I]dCTP requires a reaction time of 4 h and the percentage incorporation, when using 50 μCi, is seldom greater than 30%. After removal of unincorporated nucleotides, lyophilize the labelled DNA in an Eppendorf tube.

(ii)   Resuspend in 300 μl of hybridization fluid (50% formamide, 5 × Denhardt's solution, 5 × SSPE, 10% dextran sulphate, 200 μg/ml salmon sperm DNA) (see *Table 1* for recipes). Boil for 5 min to denature the probe and then keep on ice until use. After the tube has chilled, briefly spin in a microfuge to collect the solution at the bottom of the tube.

(iii)   Place 30 μl of hybridization mix on each slide and, using forceps, slowly lower a 22 × 50 mm coverslip from one side, taking care to avoid leaving any bubbles. Seal with rubber solution to prevent evaporation of the hybridization fluid and incubate overnight in a moist chamber at 42°C. Use the same sandwich boxes as described for the RNase step, wrapped in black plastic and floated in a water bath.

3.5 Post-hybridization washes

After hybridization, gently peel off the rubber solution without disturbing the coverslips. Remove these carefully by soaking the slides, upright, in 5 × SSC for some minutes. Transfer the slides to glass slide racks and wash in three changes of 2 × SSC at room temperature over a period of 1−2 h. The stringency of subsequent washes depends on the nature of the probe; a variety of temperatures and salt concentrations should be tried in order to find the best balance between background hybridization and specific signal. For unique sequence probes try in the range of $2 \times$ SSC at 65°C to $0.2 \times$ SSC at 60°C, for repeated sequences try $0.5-0.1 \times$ SSC at 60°C to 65°C. Stand the slides in the SSC of the selected stringencies for 1 h with one change of SSC, and follow with a wash of $0.1 \times$ SSC at room temperature for 1 h. After washing, dehydrate the slides through an alcohol series, air dry and store in a desiccator.

3.6 Dipping and developing slides

The following procedures must be carried out in the darkroom, using an appropriate safelight only when absolutely necessary. An Ilford 904 (dark brown) safelight filter is suitable for use with the Ilford Nuclear emulsion L4. The darkroom should be equipped with a water bath, set at 50°C. The emulsion is available as a shredded mousse, which can be divided into aliquots in glass jars and stored in a light-proof box. Use a glass rod to handle the mousse; never bring the emulsion into contact with any metal as this may induce background latent image.

Control slides can be informative monitors of the technique. A clean blank slide dipped in emulsion and left to expose with the rest will give an indication of any background grains present in the emulsion. A slide which has been taken through the hybridization process with unlabelled probe will indicate the level of background which the chromosome preparation itself may induce.

(i)   Dilute an aliquot of the emulsion 1:1 with distilled water and stand it in the water bath to melt. Tip the emulsion into a Coplin jar which has been pre-warmed in the water bath, stir with a glass rod and leave for 10 min to allow any air bubbles to disperse.

(ii) Dip a clean blank slide slowly in and out of the emulsion, stand it upright to drain and check under the safelight for even distribution of the emulsion layer. When the test slide is acceptable, dip the hybridized slides individually into the emulsion, allow to drain then stand them vertically in a light-proof box for 1 h whilst the emulsion dries out and hardens.

(iii) Store the slides in a light-proof box containing desiccant and leave to expose at 4°C for an appropriate period of time. Slides hybridized with repetitive and ^{125}I-labelled sequences may be ready for developing after only 2 days — try just one slide initially to judge the strength of signal. ^{3}H-labelled single copy sequences normally require 7 days or more.

(iv) Allow the slide box to warm to room temperature for 1 h before removing your slide for development. This prevents moisture condensing on the emulsion and affecting the latent image. Develop for 5 min in a solution of D19 developer (see *Table 1*) diluted 1:1 with distilled water, at 20°C. Do not agitate. Rinse in a stop bath of 1% glacial acetic acid and fix in Ilford Hypam, diluted 1:4 with water and containing Ilford Rapid Hardener, for 10 min. The hardener is essential to prevent the emulsion from swelling. Wash in very gently running water for 1 h.

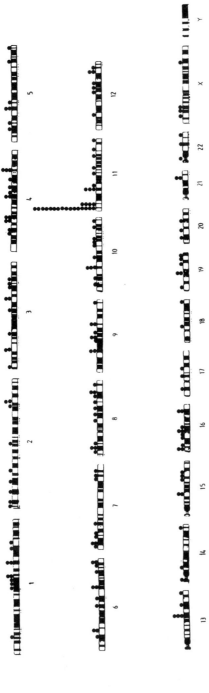

Figure 1. Distribution of silver grains observed following *in situ* hybridization of a cDNA tyrosine hydroxylase probe to human female lymphocyte chromosomes (22). The intact plasmid, which contains a 1.4-kb human coding sequence plus the pBR325 vector, was labelled by nick-translation with [^{125}I]dCTP to a specific activity of 3×10^8 d.p.m. Analysis of grain distribution in 24 cells provided a clear assignment to chromosome 11. Eleven percent of all grains scored lay in band 11p15, which comprises approximately 0.7% of the haploid human genome. Of the 20 grains scored in band 11p15, seven were clusters of more than one silver grain, which was 39% of all clusters scored.

3.7 Staining

Stain the slides in Hoescht 33258 (Sigma; B2883) diluted to 10 μg/ml in 2 × SSC for 30 min. Rinse in 2 × SSC and expose to long-wave u.v. light for 1 h as described in Section 3.2 (viii). Stain for 20 min in Giemsa diluted to 10% in pH 6.8 phosphate buffer, rinse in the same buffer and air dry.

3.8 Alternative banding techniques

In cases where BUdR incorporation during culture is not possible, chromosomes can be banded using Lipsol (19) and photographed prior to hybridization. The slides can then be de-stained, and hybridized as normal. After they have been exposed and developed, distribution of silver grains can be recorded on the previously photographed, now unbanded, spreads.

To obtain banding with the Lipsol detergent (LIP Equipment and Services Ltd., Yorkshire, UK), first place the slides in 100 volume H_2O_2, diluted 50% with water, for 3 min, rinse in methanol and air dry. Then dip in 0.5% Lipsol in pH 6.8 buffer for 10−30 sec, rinse and stain with Leishman's stain diluted 1:4 with the same buffer. Photograph good mitoses, de-stain the slides through an alcohol series and then proceed through the protocol from Section 3.3. After the slides have been developed and washed, stain in Giemsa diluted to 10% in pH 6.8 phosphate buffer for 20 min, rinse in the same buffer and air dry.

Leishman's stain is prepared by dissolving 1 g of Leishman's powder (Sigma; L6254) in 500 ml of methanol. Leave the solution at 37°C overnight and then filter.

3.9 Analysis of grain distribution

Sequences which are repeated many times at one site will give a clear signal in each cell. For single copy sequences, however, many cells need to be examined and the distribution of silver grains recorded on one ideogram in order to obtain a composite picture.

Silver grains should be scored under white light without a green filter in order to avoid confusion with spots of stain. Only score silver grains which are lying directly over, or clearly touching chromosomes. Clusters of more than one silver grain may sometimes be observed, as may separate labelling of chromatids. In both cases the grains should be scored as one hybridization event and may be depicted on the grain distribution ideograms as a large dot. Whenever the grain distribution over the whole chromosome complement is being scored, only use cells with 46 chromosomes, and with all labelled chromosomes clearly analysable. Twenty to thirty cells will normally give a clear indication of any specific signal from a unique sequence (*Figure 1*). From our own and published data, between 10 and 30% of all grains scored can be expected to be found at the specific site of hybridization. For regional localizations within a chromosome, use only cells with one or more of the relevant chromosomes labelled. Here, over 60% of grains scored should be found in one particular region of the chromosome (*Figure 2*), although the figure will vary with the length of the chromosome involved. In order to localize a sequence relative to the break point of a reciprocal translocation, the grain distributions over both translocation chromosomes and their normal homologues are required. Cells should only be used when all four chromosomes are analysable.

Cells can be photographed using Kodak Technical Pan 2415 film.

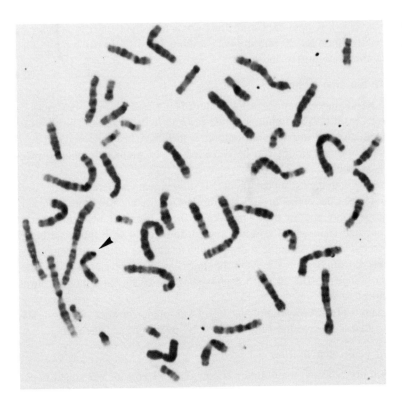

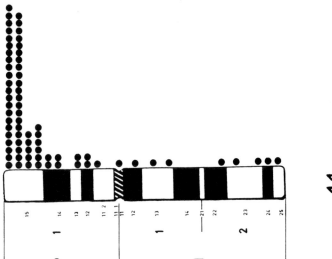

Figure 2. (a) Grain distribution on chromosome 11 in 41 cells, following *in situ* hybridization with a tyrosine hydroxylase probe (see *Figure 1* for details). Seventy one percent of cells analysed had a silver grain on one or both copies of chromosome 11. Seventy five percent of these grains were scored in band p15, and 80% of these were located toward the distal end of band p15. (b) Replication-banded female cell probed with tyrosine hydroxylase. The labelled chromosome 11 is arrowed.

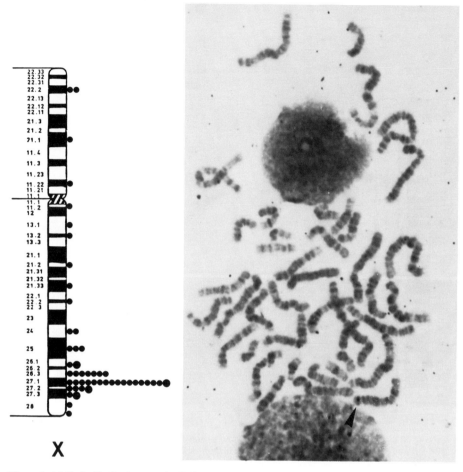

Figure 3. (a) Grain distribution over the X chromosomes in 41 cells from normal female lymphocytes, after hybridization *in situ* with the factor IX cDNA probe, which was labelled with [^{125}I]dCTP to a specific activity of 10^8 d.p.m. (23). Of the 49 grains scored, 65% lay in bands Xq26 and q27, with 35% in the proximal part of Xq27. The entire Xq27 band represents only 6% of the length of the X chromosome. (b) Replication-banded female cell probed with factor IX. The labelled active X chromosome is arrowed.

4. ALTERNATIVE DETECTION SYSTEMS

A non-radioactive detection system, sensitive enough to localize unique sequences, would be a welcome development. Burns *et al.* (20) report the use of a biotinylated probe to detect the DYZ2 repeated sequence in Y chromosome heterochromatin. They use an immunoperoxidase detection system and amplify the resultant signal by constructing a peroxidase−DAB−gold complex. This approach has been applied with some success to the localization of the globin genes (J.Jonasson, personal communication). The resolution of signal obtained by this technique should theoretically be an improvement on that obtained with radioactively labelled probes, because detection occurs directly at the site of hybridization, without the complications of an emulsion layer and electron track lengths. However, the biotin system is not yet as sensitive as the

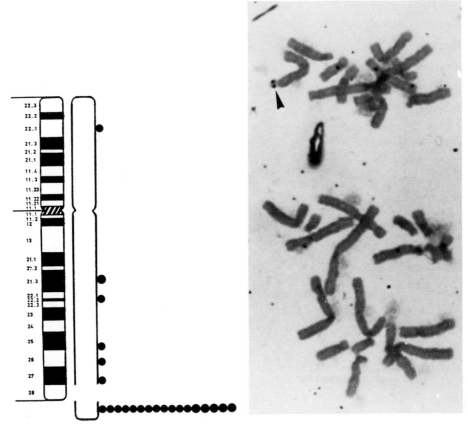

Figure 4. (a) Grain distribution over the fragile X chromosome in 20 cells obtained from a patient with fragile X mental retardation syndrome. The cells were hybridized *in situ* with a cDNA probe for factor VIIIc, which was labelled with [^{125}I]dCTP to a specific activity of 10^8 d.p.m. (23). Seventy four percent of the 23 grains scored lay distal to the fragile site, in band Xq28. (b) A fragile X chromosome labelled with factor VIIIc.

autoradiographic technique described here, and requires further improvement before it can be applied routinely to the localization of unique sequences. Another non-auto-radiographic system has been recently reported (22) using 2-acetylaminofluorine-modified probes. Again, further amplification of the detected signal is required to achieve sufficient sensitivity for localization of single copy sequences.

5. APPLICATIONS

In situ hybridization allows both repetitive and single copy sequences to be mapped within the human genome. Highest resolution in the localization of single copy sequences in our laboratory has been obtained using replication-banded normal lymphocyte chromosomes. Analysis of grain distribution directly over banded chromosomes which have been probed with a sequence from the factor IX gene (*Figure 3*) indicates that the gene lies at the proximal border of the Xq27 band in Xq27.1. The X chromosome is estimated to comprise 10^5 kb of DNA sequence and, using measurements of relative band widths

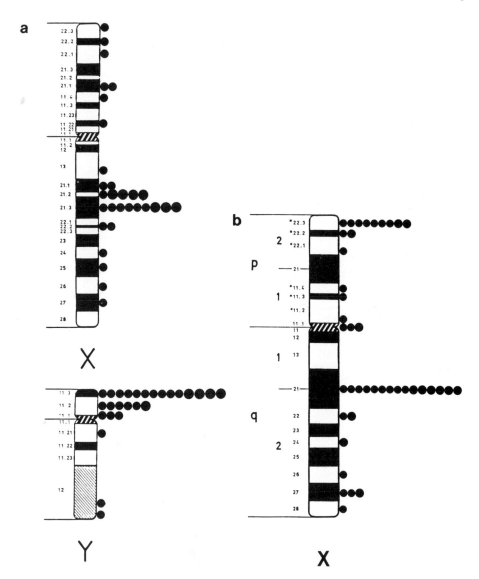

Figure 5. (a) Grain distribution over the X and Y chromosomes in 36 normal male cells probed with the X/Y homologous random DNA sequence, 75/78 (24). The sequence is assigned to Xq21 and Yp11.2-pter. **(b)** Grain distribution over the X chromosomes in 23 cells from an XX male patient. In addition to the expected signal at Xq21, another signal is present at the distal end of the short arm. This is suggested to have arisen by recombination between the X and Y short arms during the paternal meiosis.

on G-banded chromosomes (15), the band Xq27.1 can be estimated to consist of at most 5000 kb of DNA, if one assumes that the chromatin is evenly coiled. This represents the current limit of resolution of the *in situ* protocol presented here, and use of translocation break points would be expected to confirm, rather than refine, this assignment, since such distances are also approaching the limit of resolution of current cytogenetic techniques.

Structural chromosome abnormalities can, in some circumstances, prove useful for mapping purposes, particularly when ordering sequences (25,26). The structural gene for factor VIIIc can be clearly seen to be localized distal to the fragile site at Xq27.3 (*Figure 4*). Likewise, *in situ* hybridization can be a useful approach to the characterization of chromosome rearrangements. The technique has been of value in the demonstration that short arm Y chromosome material has been transferred to the short arm of one X chromosome in an 46XX male patient (*Figure 5*), and has been particularly informative in the study of the arrangement of genes around cancer-related translocation break points, in patient material and in tumour cell lines (27,28).

It seems likely that *in situ* hybridization and the approaches of molecular cytogenetics will have an increasingly important role in both the rapid assignment of cloned sequences within the genome, and the characterization of chromosomal abnormalities.

6. REFERENCES

1. Gall,J.G. and Pardue,M.L. (1969) *Proc. Natl. Acad. Sci. USA,* **63**, 378.
2. Jones,K.W. (1974) *New Techniques in Biophysics and Cell Biology,* Pain,R.H. and Smith,B.J. (eds.), John Wiley, New York, p. 29.
3. Rogers,A.W. (1979) *Techniques of Autoradiography, 3rd edn.,* Elsevier, New York.
4. Gosden,J.R., Mitchell,A.R., Buckland,A.R., Clayton,P. and Evans,H.J. (1975) *Exp. Cell Res.,* **92**, 148.
5. Chandler,M.E. and Yunis,J.J. (1978) *Cytogenet. Cell Genet.,* **22**, 352.
6. Wetmur,J.G. and Davidson,N. (1968) *J. Mol. Biol.,* **31**, 349.
7. Wahl,G.M., Stern,M. and Stark,G.R. (1979) *Proc. Natl. Acad. Sci. USA,* **76**, 3683.
8. Harper,M.E. and Saunders,G.F. (1981) *Chromosoma,* **83**, 431.
9. Evans,H.J., Buckland,R.A. and Pardue,M.L. (1974) *Chromosoma,* **48**, 405.
10. Lawrie,S.S. and Gosden,J.R. (1980) *Hum. Genet.,* **53**, 371.
11. Zabel,B.U., Naylor,S.L., Sakaguchi,A.Y., Bell,G.I. and Shows,T.B. (1983) *Proc. Natl. Acad. Sci. USA,* **80**, 6932.
12. Dutrillaux,B. and Viegas-Pequignot,E. (1981) *Hum. Genet.,* **57**, 93.
13. Shafer,D.A., Selles,W.D. and Brenner,J.F. (1982) *Am. J. Hum. Genet.,* **34**, 307.
14. Jhanwar,S.C., Burns,J.P., Alonso,M.L., Hew,W. and Chaganti,R.S.K. (1982) *Cytogenet. Cell Genet.,* **33**, 240.
15. ISCN (1981) *Cytogenet. Cell Genet.,* **31**, 1.
16. Neel,B.G., Jhanwar,S.C., Chaganti,R.S.K. and Hayward,W.S. (1982) *Proc. Natl. Acad. Sci. USA,* **79**, 7842.
17. Jhanwar,S.C., Neel,B.G., Hayward,W.S. and Chaganti,R.S.K. (1983) *Proc. Natl. Acad. Sci. USA,* **80**, 4794.
18. Chaganti,R.S.K., Jhanwar,S.C., Antonarkis,S.E. and Haywood,W.S. (1985) *Somat. Cell Mol. Genet.,* **11**, 197.
19. Stephen,G.S. (1977) *Genetics,* **47**, 115.
20. Burns,J., Chan,V.T.W., Jonasson,J.A., Fleming,K.A., Taylor,S. and McGee,J.O.D. (1985) *J. Clin. Pathol.,* **38**, 1085.
21. Landegent,J.E., Jansen in de Wal,N., Van Ommen,G.J.B., Baas,F., De Vijlder,J.J.M., Van Duijn, P. and Van der Ploeg,M. (1985) *Nature,* **317**, 175.
22. Craig,S.P., Buckle,V.J., Lamouroux,A., Mallet,J. and Craig,I.W. (1986) *Cytogenet. Cell Genet.,* in press.
23. Buckle,V.J., Craig,I.W., Hunter,D. and Edwards,J.H. (1985) *Cytogen. Cell Genet.,* **40**, 593.
24. Buckle,V.J., Boyd,Y., Craig,I.W., Fraser,N., Goodfellow,P.N. and Wolfe,J. (1985) *Cytogen. Cell. Genet.,* **40**, 593.
25. Lindgren,V., De Martinville,B., Horwich,A.L., Rosenberg,L.E. and Francke,U. (1984) *Science,* **226**, 698.
26. Morton,C.C., Kirsch,I.R., Nance,W.E., Evans,G.A., Korman,A.J. and Strominger,J.L. (1984) *Proc. Natl. Acad. Sci. USA,* **81**, 2816.
27. Le Beau,M., Diaz,M.O., Karin,M. and Rowley,J.D. (1985) *Nature,* **313**, 709.
28. Davis,M., Malcolm,S. and Rabbitts,T.H. (1984) *Nature,* **308**, 286.

CHAPTER 7

Human chromosome analysis by flow cytometry

B.D. YOUNG

1. INTRODUCTION

In recent years the application of banding techniques to the study of metaphase chromosomes has revealed many chromosomal aberrations associated with genetic disease and cancer. The cytogenetic analysis of the human karyotype is therefore of great diagnostic value and will continue to be an area of intensive study. Recent advances in recombinant DNA technology have offered the possibility of establishing the molecular nature of such abberations. The high resolution separation of human chromosomes by flow cytometry simplifies the complexity inherent in tackling such questions.

There have been many attempts to fractionate metaphase chromosomes by centrifugation, counter-current distribution and 1 *g* sedimentation. While such methods separated chromosomes from the other cellular constituents, and achieved enrichment of different size classes of chromosomes, the purification of individual chromosomes was not possible. The application of the fluorescence-activated cell sorter has allowed the purification of small but useful quantities of individual chromosomes, and therefore has become the method of choice for tackling a number of biological questions. With recombinant DNA techniques, it is now also possible to generate a large number of DNA probes for a single flow-sorted chromosome and this will prove extremely useful in the linkage analysis of certain genetic disorders.

In flow cytometry the objects to be analysed are stained in suspension with an appropriate fluorochrome and passed singly through a beam of light. The basic principles of flow analysis are shown schematically in *Figure 1*. The emitted pulses of fluorescence are measured and stored in the form of a histogram of the number of pulses versus fluorescence intensity. Thus any population of cellular objects that can be made sufficiently fluorescent can be analysed in this way. Gray *et al.* (1,2) first analysed Chinese hamster metaphase chromosomes by flow cytometry after staining with ethidium bromide and obtained a characteristic series of peaks. This was later extended to human chromosomes, and other fluorochromes were introduced (3,4). It was clear from such experiments that flow cytometry could be used to sort certain human chromosomes with a high level of purity, the only disadvantage being the relatively small amount of material obtained (e.g. 10^6 average-sized human chromosomes is equivalent to about 250 ng of DNA).

PRINCIPLE OF CELL SORTING

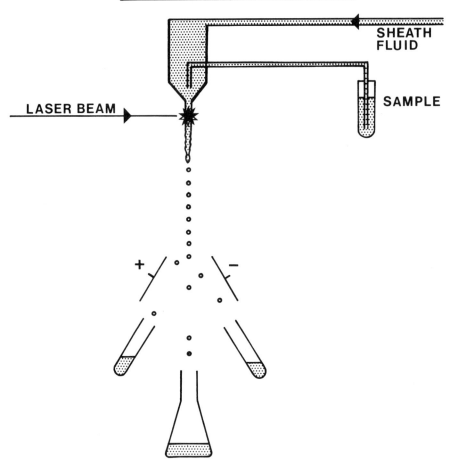

Figure 1. Schematic diagram showing the principles of flow analysis and sorting.

2. TECHNICAL CONSIDERATIONS

2.1 Preparative techniques

Although several different approaches have been developed over the last few years, they all have certain common features. A culture of growing cells is usually treated with an agent such as colcemid or vinblastine in order to arrest sufficient cells in metaphase. The period of treatment may depend on the cell cycle time, but extensive culture in the presence of such agents can lead to a high degree of chromosome contraction. If the cells grow as an attached layer, mitotic shake-off can be used to obtain an enriched population of metaphase cells. However, suspension cell lines may also be used if sufficient metaphase cells are present and if care is taken not to lyse nuclei of the interphase cells which predominate in the population. The cell population is then usually subjected to hypotonic swelling and treated with a detergent. The next step is

Table 1. Chromosome preparation for flow cytometry.

pH	Detergent	Lysis	Stabilizing agent	Fluorochrome	References
7.5	–	S	Hexylene glycol	EB	(1,2,6)
7.5	Triton X	S	Mg^{2+}	EB + M	(42)
7.2	Digitonin	V	Polyamines	EB	(8)
–	–	V	PI	PI	(14)
–	Triton X	S	Psoralen (AMT)	Hoechst 33258	(12)
–	Triton X	S	PI	PI	(13)
1% Acetic acid	–	U	Hexylene glycol	DAPI	(16)
7.5	Triton X	S	Mg^{2+}	PI	(5)
8.0	–	S	Mg^{2+}	PI, Hoechst 33258	(19)

S = syringe; V = vortexing; U = ultrasound; EB = ethidium bromide; PI = propidium iodide; M = mithramycin.

to lyse the mitotic cells by mechanical disruption such as passage through a fine needle or by vigorous vortexing. During the lysis process it is helpful to monitor the disruption of the mitotic cells on a fluorescence or phase contrast microscope, since insufficient treatment will not lyse sufficient cells or disrupt chromosome clumps whereas excessive treatment can cause chromosome breakage. Differential centrifugation may then be used to remove interphase nuclei, if present.

The high resolution offered by flow cytometry has led to increasing interest in the optimization of the bulk preparation of chromosomes. The ideal technique would optimize cell lysis and minimize chromosome damage. However, as there is no clear agreement among investigators on the best technique for preparing chromosomes for flow analysis, all the methods used have been summarized in *Table 1*. When deciding which method to adopt, it should be borne in mind that the different methods may be optimal for different cell types, as suggested by Bijman (5).

The first flow karyotype analyses (1,2,6) were obtained using the hexylene glycol procedure of Wray and Stubblefield (7). This approach has the advantage that the banding structure of chromosomes is sufficiently preserved to allow direct analysis of chromosomes after sorting. Carrano *et al.* (3) investigated the influence of several factors on this protocol, such as shearing forces and cell concentration. Also the addition of sodium dodecyl sulphate, ribonuclease and trypsin were found to have a negative effect. An alternative approach for the bulk isolation of chromosomes using polyamines to stabilize the DNA was developed for flow analysis by Sillar and Young (8) from the method of Blumethal *et al.* (9). A direct comparison of the two methods using the same Chinese hamster ovary (CHO) cell culture indicated that the polyamine method yielded lower background levels and superior coefficients of variation. A disadvantage of this method is that the highly condensed state of the chromosomes prevents direct banding studies on sorted chromosomes. However, quinacrine studies on sorted chromosomes prepared in this way have been described (10). This technique has been used successfully in our laboratory on a variety of cell lines and peripheral blood samples and is summarised in *Table 2*. A comparative study (11), which did not include flow analysis, concluded that the polyamine method of Blumethal *et al.* (9) was more appropriate than the hexylene glycol-based method as judged by micrococcal nuclease digestion of the chromosomal DNA. Yu *et al.* (12) investigated the use of 4'-aminomethyl-4,5',8-tri-

Table 2. This method (8) is based on that described by Blumenthal *et al.* (9) in which the polyamines, spermine and spermidine are used to stabilize the chromosomes and the detergent digitonin is used to assist cell lysis. This method has been used as the preparation technique prior to flow sorting by a number of workers and in our laboratory we have found it to be the most satisfactory.

1. Treat cells with 0.032 μg/ml of colcemid for 5 – 16 h, depending on the rate of cell growth.
2. Harvest mitotic cells by gentle shaking of the culture flasks.
3. Centrifuge at 800 r.p.m. for 10 min.
4. Discard the supernatant and resuspend in 0.075 M KCl at 4°C for 30 min in order to swell the cells.
5. Centrifuge at 300 r.p.m. for 15 min.
6. Discard the supernatant and resuspend the pellet in isolation buffer (15 mM Tris-HCl, 0.2 mM spermine, 0.5 mM spermidine, 2 mM EDTA, 0.5 mM EGTA, 80 mM KCl, 20 mM NaCl, 14 mM β-mercaptoethanol, pH 7.2).
7. Centrifuge at 1500 r.p.m. for 2 min.
8. Repeat steps 6 and 7.
9. Resuspend the final pellet in approximately 20 times its volume of ice-cold isolation buffer containing 0.1% digitonin. Digitonin is dissolved just prior to use by warming to 37°C and filtering out any insoluble materials.
10. The final volume, typically 2 ml, is agitated vigorously for 1 min on a vortex mixer.
11. The lysis of metaphase cells should be monitored by fluorescence or phase contrast microscopy.

methylpsoralen to stabilize the chromosomes, but their data did not indicate that this method was superior to the hexylene glycol method.

The use of the intercalating fluorochrome propidium iodide to stabilize chromosome structure has been investigated by Buys *et al.* (12). It was demonstrated that chromosomes isolated in this way maintained their banding structure. A similar protocol but with 0.1% sodium citrate and the addition of ethanol to 20% prior to lysis has been reported by Matsson and Rydberg (14). This method is based on that developed by Krishan (15) for staining human lymphoblasts, and was claimed to cause less damage to interphase cell nuclei than other methods. Stoehr *et al.* (16) have reported a hexylene glycol-based protocol which involves mild fixation with 1% acetic acid and sonication to disrupt the mitotic cells. Although acidic treatment (50% acetic acid) was shown by Tien Kuo (11) to result in extensive damage to the chromosomal DNA, it was claimed the relatively mild treatment in this protocol would not prevent DNA analysis on sorted chromosomes. A low pH protocol has been devised by Collard *et al.* (17) for the velocity sedimentation of chromosomes followed by flow analysis. Mitotic cells are lysed in the presence of 2% citric acid which gives superior resolving power on 1 *g* sedimentation. However, since chromosomes sedimented at low pH are not suitable for DNA analysis, Collard *et al.* (18) have subsequently modified the sucrose gradient to neutral pH.

A comparative study of the influence of several ions and detergents has been reported by Bijman (5). The optimal chromosome buffer contained magnesium (3 – 5 mM), sodium (10 mM), Tris (10 mM) and Triton X-100 (0.4%) as judged by flow analysis. Magnesium ions were found to be necessary for the stability of the chromosomes, whereas sodium and potassium had no effect, with calcium having a negative effect. Van den Engh *et al.* (19) have described an isolation buffer at pH 8.0 which uses $MgSO_4$ to stabilize the chromosomes. Another feature of this method is the use of RNase to reduce the background fluorescence due to binding of fluorochromes to RNA. It has recently been reported that the addition of sodium citrate to 10 mM can improve the resolution obtainable by this method (20).

2.2 **Choice of DNA-specific stain**

There are several criteria which a DNA-specific stain must fulfil if it is to be useful in flow cytometry. Firstly, the wavelength of excitation must match the available light source. Most flow instruments use laser illumination and have a restricted set of output wavelengths in the range 458 − 514 nm, and also a u.v. output at 360 nm. The relatively small DNA content of most chromsomes requires that the chosen stain has the highest possible quantum efficiency. This is important in reducing statistical errors in measurement of chromosomal fluorescence. Also, the stain should be insensitive to the degree of chromosomal contraction which can be quite variable in a chromosomal preparation. The specificities and characteristics of DNA-binding fluorochromes are summarized in *Table 3*.

The first flow karyotypes were obained using ethidium bromide as a DNA-specific stain (1,2,6), and this has remained one of the principal stains used. Jensen *et al.* (21) investigated the suitability of ethidium bromide, Hoechst 33258 and chromomycin A_3 for flow analysis of chromosomes and demonstrated that both Hoechst 33258 and chromomycin A_3 yielded flow karyotypes with distinct differences from that obtained with ethidium bromide. It has been shown that Hoechst 33258 has an AT-binding preference, (22) chromomycin A_3 has a GC-binding preference (23) and ethidium bromide has no base sequence preference (24). It has therefore been concluded that the differences observed with such stains are due to differences in chromosomal base composition or accessibility. A comparative study of the use of ethidium bromide, Hoechst 33258, chromomycin A_3, 4′,6-diamidino-2-phenylindole acid (DAPI) and propidium iodide for flow cytometry of metaphase chromosomes has been reported by Langlois *et al.* (25). DAPI binds preferentially to AT-rich DNA and the relative intensities of DAPI-stained chromosomes are similar to Hoechst 33258-stained chromosomes. Similarly, propidium iodide, which is not thought to have a base preference, yields profiles which are similar to those obtained using ethidium bromide. It was also shown by analysis of double-stained chromosomes that bound stains interact by energy transfer with little or no binding competition.

Table 3. Nucleic acid fluorochromes for flow cytometry.

Name	Excitation (nm)[a]	Emission (nm)[b]	Specificity (pH 7)[c]
DAPI	365 (or 351/364)	415−520 (460)	DNA/(RNA)
Hoechst 33342	365 (or 351/364)	425−520 (465)	DNA (A=T)
Mithramycin	434 (or 457)	500−630 (565)	DNA (G = C)
Chromomycin	434 (or 457)	490−625 (555)	DNA (G = C)
Thioflavin T	434 (or 457)	470−530 (490)	Single strand NA
Acridine orange	488	535/>600	Polycations
Ethidium bromide	488	570−645 (605)	Double strand NA
Propidium bromide	488 (or 546)	580−660 (620)	Double strand NA
Pyronin Y	546 (or 514)	570−605 (580)	RNA (DNA)
7 NH$_2$-AMD	546 (or 514)	610−700 (655)	DNA (G = C)

[a]Excitation wavelengths are those available in commercial flow cytometers.
[b]Emission data gives the wavelength range for half-maximum, and the maximum.
[c]Specificity includes both binding and fluorescence enhancement.
NA = nucleic acid.
Reproduced by permission of Dr James Gill, Becton Dickinson.

Conventional fluorescence microscopy was used by Latt *et al.* (26) to study interactions between a number of DNA-binding dyes on metaphase chromosomes. It was shown that if the energy acceptor dye (e.g. actinomycin D or Methyl green) has a binding specificity opposite to the binding of fluorescence specificity of the donor (e.g. Hoechst 33258, quinacrine or chromomycin A_3) contrast in donor fluorescence can be enhanced, leading to patterns selectively highlighting standard or reverse chromosome bands. Recently the counterstaining of human chromosomes with the non-fluorescent AT-specific DNA-binding agent, netropsin, has been used in flow analysis (27). The use of netropsin alters the fluorescence signal from the C-band heterochromatin of certain human chromosomes and thus can enhance their resolution from other chromosomes. In a similar manner an abnormal human chromosome 15 was identified by counter-staining with either netropsin or distamycin A (28).

2.3 Alternative methods for fluorescent labelling of chromosomes

The use of monoclonal antibodies against chromosomal proteins provides an alternative method for labelling chromosomes. Chromosome suspensions were treated with a mouse monoclonal antibody specific for histone 2B followed by fluoresceinated goat anti-mouse IgM antibody (29). Although the binding of anti-H2B was proportional to DNA content the resolution in flow was inferior to that obtained with a DNA-specific fluorochrome. The main application of this approach may be to allow the study of chromosome structure by flow cytometry.

A possible approach for labelling specific chromosomes is the use of *in situ* hybridization of biotinylated DNA probes to suspensions of chromosomes. The fluorescent detection of the hybridized probe can be obtained with an avidin − fluorochrome conjugate. This approach has already been reported for chromosomes fixed on slides (30) and could allow the fluorescent labelling of specific chromosomes or parts of chromosomes for flow analysis. However, it has yet to be demonstrated that hybridization can be obtained on chromosomes in suspension.

2.4 Technical innovation

The quality of flow karyotype analysis is critically dependent on the resolving power of the machine used. Much effort has gone into technical improvement and innovation in order to obtain superior analysis. Conventional machines measure the fluorescence emitted by each chromosome in terms of pulse height or area. However, Cram *et al.* (31) found pulse width to be a good parameter for resolving chromosomes as a function of total emission in the case of the smaller chromosomes, and orientation (i.e. arm length) for larger chromosomes. A novel method which is based on chromosome structure rather than simply DNA content, is based on the principle that certain chromosomes will orientate in the direction of flow. Therefore, as each chromosome passes a narrow window, a fluorescence signal along the length of the chromosome, with a pronounced drop at the centromere, should be obtained. Such profiles have been obtained from the Indian muntjac No. 1 chromosome (32) and from certain Chinese hamster chromosomes (33), and the centrometric indices thus calculated were found to be in good agreement with the values obtained by conventional microscopic measurement. Although this approach has the capability of identifying uniquely the larger chromosomes in flow, it has so far been unable to analyse chromosomes which are too small to orientate in the sample stream.

One of the most promising innovations, particularly for the analysis of human chromosomes, has been the introduction of dual beam flow cytometry. Chromosomes are double stained with Hoechst 33258 and chromomycin A_3, each of which is excited independently, and the resultant fluorescence values are presented as correlated two parameter analysis. It has been demonstrated that the Hoechst 33258 and the chromomycin A_3 fluorescence can each be measured almost independently (34). With this technique it has been possible to resolve all the human chromosomes, with the exception of Nos. 9 − 12 and 14,15 (35). A disadvantage of this approach for its general application is that, currently, expensive laser light sources are required.

Recently, high resolution of Chinese hamster chromosomes has been reported (35), using a specially designed flow cytometer to achieve high illumination irradiance. It was possible to achieve 10 times greater irradiance than in most other machines. As a result, the fluorescence from metaphase chromosomes was less dependent on laser power, with a doubling of power from 1 to 2 W producing only a 15% increase in signal.

3. APPLICATIONS OF CHROMOSOME FRACTIONATION

3.1 Flow karyotype analysis

With current techniques and equipment it is possible to measure the fluorescence of human chromosomes with coefficients of variation of $1 - 2\%$. At such a level of resolution many of the human chromosomes can be individually resolved, and it has therefore become possible to quantitate accurately the DNA content in both normal and abnormal karyotypes. A series of flow karyotypes is shown in *Figure 2*, in which the numbers indicate which chromosomes correspond to each peak. These developments have, for the first time, opened up the possibility of using flow cytometry to provide routine karyotype analysis. In order to investigate the feasibility of such an application, we have applied flow cytometry (37) to chromosomes prepared from a series of human peripheral blood samples. It was shown that the slight variations in these flow karyotypes could be attributed to polymorphic heterochromatin at the centromeres of certain chromosomes (arrowed in *Figure 2*). An extensive study (38) has shown that certain chromosomes are relatively invariant in DNA content, whilst others such as 1, 9, 16 and Y chromosomes can vary considerably in DNA content in normal individuals. Clearly, before flow cytometry can be fully developed to provide automated analysis of the human karyotype, it will be necessary to take account of these normally occurring polymorphisms. One approach might be to suppress the fluorescence from the heterochromatic regions using an agent like netropsin as described by Meyne *et al.* (24).

The effect of certain chromosomal abnormalities on the flow karyotype can be predicted. For example, a trisomy should be detected as a 50% increase in the area of the peak corresponding to that chromosome. Translocations which result in a net change in DNA content should be detected by the presence of the chromosomes involved in an abnormal position in the profile. Recently, Wirchubsky *et al.* (39) have applied flow analysis to a series of cell lines bearing translocations associated with Burkitt's lymphoma. In particular the $14q^+$ chromosome in the t(8;14), the $2p^-$ in the t(2;8) and the $22q^-$ in the t(8;22) could be separately identified by flow analysis.

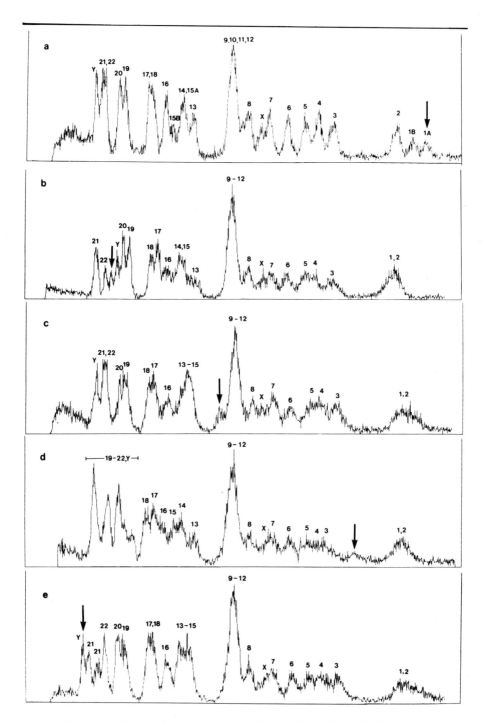

Figure 2. A series of flow karyotypes from normal individuals. The position of each chromosome is indicated and the polymorphic variations are arrowed.

This approach has recently been extended to murine plasmacytomas (40).

Flow cytometry has also proven useful in assessing chromosomal changes occuring in experimental systems. Karyotype changes have long been observed in spontaneously transformed Chinese hamster embryo fibroblasts, and Cram *et al.* (41) have used conventional banding studies and high resolution flow cytometry to analyse in detail such progressive changes. One of the earliest changes, which preceded tumorigenicity in nude mice, was the occurrence of a trisomy of chromosome 5. A steady progression in karyotype instability was observed, corresponding to neoplastic evolution of these cells.

Flow analysis can also be used to monitor random karyotype changes induced by mutagenic agents. The clastogenic effect of chemical mutagens and X rays on Chinese hamster chromosomes was monitored using flow analysis by Otto and Oldiges (42). Such agents cause random damage to chromosomes and therefore result in the broadening of the peaks in a profile. The clastogenic effectiveness of such agents was quantified, and the dose-effect relationship was established by the increase of the coefficient of variation of the peak of the largest chromosomes type in the flow histogram. Green *et al.* (42) have shown that the effect of *in vitro* radiation doses on human peripheral blood lymphocytes can be successfully monitored by flow analysis of chromosome damage.

It should be emphasized that there are certain karyotype changes which would be undetectable by flow cytometry. For example, a reciprocal translocation in which equal amounts of DNA were exchanged would have no effect on the flow karyotype. For this reason, flow cytometry is best used in conjunction with conventional banding studies to provide accurate quantitative data on karyotype changes.

3.2 Gene mapping using flow-sorted chromosomes

The application of flow cytometry to chromosomal analysis is greatly enhanced by the sorting facility provided on most machines. It has been possible to identify chromosomes in flow karyotypes by sorting each fraction and performing banding studies. This has been done for the Chinese hamster (1), the Indian muntjac (44) and the human karyotype (3). The purity of the Chinese hamster fractions ranged from 95% pure chromosome 1 to 76% pure chromosomes 9 and M1. Such levels of purity are considerably better than those achieved by other fractionation procedures. However, a limitation of flow sorting as a preparative procedure is the amount of material which can be sorted in a reasonable period of time (e.g. 10^6 average sized human chromosome equals about 250 ng of DNA). This limation can be overcome by pre-enrichment of chromosomes by centrifugation (18,45). Alternatively the biochemical techniques applied to sorted chromosomes can be modified to deal with such small quantities.

The application of restriction enzyme digestion and Southern analysis to the DNA of sorted chromosomes has permitted the mapping of certain genes. Lebo *et al.* (45) assigned members of the human globin gene family to the short arm of chromosome 11 by flow sorting of chromosomes from normal cells and from cells bearing translocations of chromosome 11. Similarly, Lebo *et al.* (47) mapped the insulin gene to the short arm of chromosome 11. Random DNA probes were mapped on chromosome 22 by flow sorting and probing translocations of 22 (48). Collard *et al.* (49) used an alternative approach by pre-enriching rat chromosomes by velocity sedimentation. The individual fractions were characterized by flow cytometry and the rat kappa light chain immunoglobulin and the rat albumin genes were mapped by molecular hybridisation. The application of chromosome sorting to gene mapping has been extensively reviewed by Lebo (50). Collard *et al.* (51) have recently described single copy gene mapping with as little as 10 000 − 30 000 chromosomes sorted directly on to nitrocellulose.

3.3 **Chromosomal DNA library construction**

There are a number of genetic diseases which have a chromosomal assignment but an unknown biochemical basis. The molecular study of these conditions can be greatly enhanced if a source of DNA fragments is available for the chromosome in question. Hence the construction of DNA libraries enriched by flow sorting for single human chromosomes is an area of considerable interest. Having constructed such a library, it is important to assess its degree of purity. The most complete way of assessing purity is to pick at random a number of single copy clones and to map them, by molecular hybridization to further sorted chromosomes or to DNA of a cell hybrid panel.

A number of chromosome-enriched DNA libraries have now been constructed. Phage vectors have been used in these constructions because their superior cloning efficiency is necessary for the relatively small amounts of sorted chromosomal DNA available. For the same reason, most libraries represent complete rather than partial enzyme digests. Complete digestion implies that certain DNA fragments will be too small or large to be represented in a library. Hence partial digestion, though difficult to achieve, is preferable (52). Using the preparative procedure described in *Table 1*, we have constructed a series of chromosome-specific libraries: chromosome X (53), chromosomes 21, 22 (48), chromosome 6 (52). The chromosome 22 library has been used for the cloning of a human Vλ immunoglobulin gene (54) and the chromosome 6 library used for the cloning of a series of HLA clones. The use of such enriched libraries had the advantages that the possibility of cloning pseudo-genes was greatly reduced and that a smaller number of recombinant phages had to be screened. A program for the sorting and cloning of all the human chromosomes has recently been undertaken by the laboratories of Los Alamos and Livermore. The availability of these libraries will greatly enhance the molecular analysis of genetic disease.

A number of human tumours exhibit homogeneously staining chromosomal regions (HSR), which represent amplification of certain DNA sequences. The presence of such a region of a human chromosome 1, increasing its DNA content by about 50%, allowed Kanda *et al.* (55) to flow-sort this chromosome from its normal homologue and to construct a DNA library. From this library it was possible to isolate DNA clones which mapped by *in situ* hybridization to the HSR on chromosome 1. This illustrates the possibility of using chromosomal aberrations to separate chromosomes which cannot otherwise be resolved. The presence of abnormal amounts of centric heterochromatin in a chromosome may also prove useful in this regard (38).

4. REFERENCES

1. Gray,J.W., Carrano,A.V., Steinmetz,L.L., Van Dilla,M.A., Moore,D.H.,II, Mayall,B.H. and Mendelsohn,M.L. (1975) *Proc. Natl. Acad. Sci. USA*, **72**, 1231.

2. Gray,J.W., Carrano,A.V., Moore,D.H.,II, Steinmetz,L.L., Minkler,J., Mayall,B.H., Mendelsohn,M.L. and Van Dilla,M.A. (1975) *Clin. Chem.*, **21**, 1258.
3. Carrano,A.V., Van Dilla,M.A. and Gray,J.W. (1979) In *Flow Cytometry and Sorting*, Melamed,M., Mullaney,P.F. and Mendelsohn,M.L. (eds), John Wiley and Sons, New York, p. 421.
4. Carrano,A.V., Gray,J.W., Langlois,R.G., Burkhart-Schultz,K.J. and Van Dilla,M.A. (1979) *Proc. Natl. Acad. Sci. USA*, **76**, 1382.
5. Bijman,Th.J. (1983) *Cytometry*, **3**, 354.
6. Stubblefield,E., Cram,S. and Deaven,L. (1975) *Exp. Cell. Res.*, **94**, 464.
7. Wray,W. and Stubblefield,E. (1970) *Exp. Cell Res.*, **59**, 469.
8. Sillar,R. and Young,B.D. (1981) *J. Histochem. Cytochem.*, **29**, 74.
9. Blumenthal,A.B., Dieden,J.D., Kapp,L.N. and Sedat,J.W. (1979) *J. Cell Biol.*, **81**, 255.
10. Fantes,J.A., Green,D.K. and Cooke,H.J. (1983) *Cytometry*, **4**, 88.
11. Tien Kuo,M. (1982) *Exp. Cell Res.*, **138**, 221.
12. Yu,L.C., Aten,J., Gray,J. and Carrano,A.V. (1981) *Nature*, **293**, 154.
13. Buys,C.H.C.M., Koerts,T. and Aten,J.A. (1982) *Hum. Genet.*, **61**, 157.
14. Matsson,P. and Rydberg,B. (1981) *Cytometry*, **1**, 369.
15. Krishan,A. (1977) *Stain Technol.*, **52**, 339.
16. Stoehr,M., Hutter,K.J., Frank,M. and Goerttler,K. (1982) *Histochemistry*, **74**, 57.
17. Collard,J.G., Tulp,A., Stegeman,J., Boezeman,J., Bauer,F.W., Jongkind,J.F. and Verkerk,A. (1980) *Exp. Cell Res.*, **130**, 217.
18. Collard,J.G., Tulp,A., Stegeman,J. and Boezeman,J. (1981) *Exp. Cell Res.*, **133**, 341.
19. Van den Engh,G., Trask,B., Cram,S. and Bartholdi,M. (1984) *Cytometry*, **5**, 108.
20. Van den Engh,G.J., Trask,B., Gray,J.W., Langlois,R.G. and Yu,L.C. (1985) *Cytometry*, **6**, 92.
21. Jensen,R.H., Langlois,R.G. and Mayall,B.H. (1977) *J. Histochem. Cytochem.*, **25**, 954.
22. Latt,S.A. and Wohlleb,J. (1975) *Chromosoma*, **52**, 2973.
23. Behr,W., Honikel,K. and Hartmann,G. (1969) *Eur. J. Biochem.*, **9**, 82.
24. Le Pecq,J.B. and Paoletti,C. (1967) *J. Mol. Biol.*, **27**, 87.
25. Langlois,R.G., Carrano,A.V., Gray,J.W. and Van Dilla,M.A. (1980) *Chromosoma*, **77**, 229.
26. Latt,S.A., Sahar,E., Eisenhard,M.E. and Juergens,L.A. (1980) *Cytometry*, **1**, 2.
27. Meyne,J., Bartholdi,M., Travis,G. and Cram,L.S. (1984) *Cytometry*, **5**, 580.
28. Lalande,M., Schreck,R.R., Hoffman,R. and Latt,S.A. (1985) *Cytometry*, **6**, 1.
29. Trask,B., van den Engh,G., Gray,J., Vanderlaan,M. and Turner,B. (1984) *Chromosoma*, **90**, 295.
30. Lau,Y.F. (1985) *Cytogenet. Cell Genet.*, **39**, 184.
31. Cram,L.S., Arndt-Jovin,D.J., Grimwade,B.G. and Jovin,T. (1979) *J. Histochem. Cytochem.*, **27**, 445.
32. Gray,J.W., Peters,D., Merrill,J.T., Martin,R. and Van Dilla,M.A. (1979) *J. Histochem. Cytochem.*, **27**, 441.
33. Gray,J.W., Lucas,J., Pinkel,D., Peters,D., Ashworth,L. and Van Dilla,M.A. (1980) *Flow Cytometry IV*, Universitetsforlaget, Norway, p. 249.
34. Gray,J.W., Langlois,R.G., Carrano,A.V., Burkhart-Schultz,K. and Van Dilla,M.A. (1979) *Chromosoma (Berl.)*, **73**, 9.
35. Langlois,R.G., Yu,L.C., Gray,J.W. and Carrano,A.V. (1982) *Proc. Natl. Acad. Sci. USA*, **79**, 7876.
36. Bartholdi,M.F., Sinclair,D.C. and Cram,L.S. (1983) *Cytometry*, **3**, 395.
37. Young,B.D., Ferguson-Smith,M.A., Sillar,R. and Boyd,E. (1981) *Proc. Natl. Acad. Sci. USA*, **78**, 7727.
38. Harris,P., Boyd,E., Young,B.D. and Ferguson-Smith,M.A. (1985) *Cell Genet. Cytogenet.*, in press.
39. Wirchubsky,Z., Perlmann,C., Lindsten,J. and Klein,G. (1983) *Int. J. Cancer*, **32**, 147.
40. Wirchubsky,Z., Weiner,F., Spira,J., Sumegi,J., Perlmann,C. and Klein,G. (1984) *Cancer Cells/Oncogenes and Viral Genes*, **2**, 253.
41. Cram,L.S., Bartholdi,M.F., Ray,F.A., Travis,G.L. and Kraemer,P.M. (1983) *Cancer Res.*, **43**, 4828.
42. Otto,F.J. and Oldiges,H. (1980) *Cytometry*, **1**, 13.
43. Green,D.K., Fantes,J.A. and Spowart,G. (1984) In *Biological Dosimetry*, Eisert,W.G. and Mendelsohn,M.L. (eds.), Springer-Verlag, Berlin, p. 6
44. Carrano,A.V., Gray,J.W., Moore,D.H., Minkler,J.L., Mayall,B.H., Van Dilla,M.A. and Mendelsohn,M.L. (1976) *J. Histochem. Cytochem.*, **24**, 348.
45. Stubblefield,E. and Oro,J. (1982) *Cytometry*, **2**, 273.
46. Lebo,R.V., Carrano,A.V., Burkhart-Schultz,K.J., Dozy,A.M., Yu,L.C. and Kan,Y.W. (1979) *Proc. Natl. Acad. Sci. USA*, **76**, 5804.
47. Lebo,R.V., Kan,Y.W., Cheung,M.C., Carrano,A.V., Yu,L.C., Chang,J.C., Cordell,B. and Goodman,H.M. (1982) *Hum. Genet.*, **60**, 10.
48. Krumlauf,R., Jeanpierre,M. and Young,B.D. (1982) *Proc. Natl. Acad. Sci. USA*, **79**, 2971.
49. Collard,J.G., Schijven,J., Tulp,A. and Meulenbrook,M. (1982) *Exp. Cell Res.*, **137**, 463.

111

50. Lebo,R. (1982) *Cytometry*, **3**, 145.
51. Collard,J.G., de Boer,P.A.J., Janssen,J.W.G., Schijven,J.F. and de Jong,B. (1985) *Cytometry*, **6**, 179.
52. Boncinelli,E., Goyns,M.H., Scotto,L., Simeone,A., Harris,P., Kellow,J.E. and Young,B.D. (1984) *Mol. Biol. Med.*, **2**, 1.
53. Davies,K.E., Young,B.D., Elles,R.G., Hill,M.E. and Williamson,R. (1981) *Nature*, **293**, 374.
54. Anderson,M.L.M., Szajnert,M.F., Kaplan,J.C., McColl,L. and Young,B.D. (1984) *Nucleic Acids Res.*, **12**, 6647.
55. Kanda,N., Schreck,R., Alt,F., Bruns,G., Baltimore,D. and Latt,S.A. (1977) *Proc. Natl. Acad. Sci. USA*, **80**, 4069.

CHAPTER 8

Restriction analysis of chromosomal DNA in a size range up to two million base pairs by pulsed field gradient electrophoresis

G.J.B. VAN OMMEN and J.M.H. VERKERK

1. INTRODUCTION

In present day molecular biology, the upper size limit to continuous stretches of DNA which can be cloned and studied with reasonable effort lies around 100−150 kb. This corresponds to a few chromosome walking steps with a cosmid cloning system, the highest capacity cloning system presently available (see Chapter 5). Due to the cosmid insert size of 35−45 kb, a first screening with a single-copy genomic DNA probe usually yields a set of clones overlapping 35−70 kb. Subsequent steps with subcloned unique probes located near the edges of the cloned segment allow an outward progress of 20−30 kb in each subsequent step. Using cDNA as starting probe, one might fortuitously obtain clones covering a larger region, when the gene of interest contains many large introns. A striking example of this is the human thyroglobulin gene, located near the end of the long arm of chromosome 8 (distal to c-*myc*), of which thusfar 300 kb of genomic clones have been obtained, including a giant intron of 64 kb (1,2 and F.Baas and G.J.B.van Ommen, manuscript in preparation). In the case of a clustering of many homologous genes a more extensive chromosome walk is feasible because the probe simultaneously detects many adjacent regions. By this means, chromosomal regions of about 1000 kb around both the mouse H2 locus and its human MHC counterpart have been opened up for further study (3,4).

These cases are exceptional however, and the development of techniques permitting a systematic study of chromosomal regions covering several hundreds or thousands of kilobase pairs has been much awaited by the human geneticist to address questions regarding, amongst others, chromosomal instability, translocations, amplifications and a vast potential of minor chromosomal aberrations which fall below the resolution of the light microscope.

One example of the application of such techniques can be found in the molecular analysis of Duchenne muscular dystrophy (DMD) (5), located in the middle of the short arm of the X-chromosome, in band Xp21 (6). This crippling and eventually fatal neuro-muscular disease has an incidence of about 1:3300 males and the highest known spontaneous mutation rate, around 1:10 000 (7). It has therefore been speculated that the DMD region might contain features conferring an unusual instability upon this area (8). Consistent with this, around 10 cases of DMD in females have been described, all caused by balanced Xp21-autosomal translocations (e.g. 9), which leads to preferential inactivation of the normal X-chromosome.

We have recently isolated a cloned DNA fragment, called 754, which maps physically and genetically close to the DMD locus (10). It maps into a minor interstitial deletion of the central part of Xp21 in a male affected amongst other disorders by DMD (11). The deletion is estimated to cover 6×10^6 bp. The genetic linkage between DMD and a restriction fragment length polymorphism (RFLP) detected by 754 also suggests that 754 maps at most a few million base pairs from the DMD locus. Thus, 754 provides a foothold in the vicinity of DMD, to be used for chromosome walking or jumping to the locus itself. To get some idea of the actual distances involved, the method of pulsed field gradient (PFG) electrophoresis can be applied.

The PFG electrophoresis technique was originally developed by Schwarz and Cantor (12) and modified by Carle and Olson (13). This technique allows resolution of DNA fragments up to about 2×10^6 bp (2Mb). The construction of a restriction map on this scale around 754 and other Xp21 probes, and the comparison of maps of normal individuals and translocation and deletion patients, should allow us to get a more precise idea of the DNA rearrangements involved.

This application of PFG electrophoresis to DMD was prompted by the rapid progress of deletion analysis around the DMD locus (11,14,15). However, many other applications of this technique can be envisaged. This chapter deals more in general with setting up the electrophoresis system, the preparation of marker DNA sets, an application to restriction digestion and blot hybridization of mammalian DNA using single-copy probes, including some problems encountered and their possible solutions. Besides technical aspects, such as the choice of enzymes, the discussion covers some of the ideas on the background of the PFG method and several potential applications. The reader should bear in mind, however, that the technique is still very much 'state of the art', so that major improvements and new applications are likely to evolve in the near future.

2. MATERIALS AND METHODS

2.1 Preparation of agarose blocks containing human DNA

White blood cells are obtained by isotonic lysis of whole blood (10). Tissue culture cells are collected using standard procedures.

(i)   Wash the cells once in SE (75 mM NaCl, 25 mM Na-EDTA, pH 7.4) and resuspend in SE at 30×10^6 cells/ml, at room temperature.

(ii)   Melt 1% LGT agarose (Biorad) in SE, cool to about 50°C and mix in a 1:1 ratio with the cell suspension.

(iii) Immediately dispense the mixture into slots of $10 \times 6 \times 1.5$ mm, made through a Perspex mould (see *Figure 1*) and cover on one side with tape.

(iv)   Put the mould on ice for 5−10 min.

(v)   Remove the tape and blow the solidified blocks gently out of the slots using a Pasteur pipette balloon.

(vi)   Collect the blocks in about five volumes of ES (0.5 M EDTA, 1% Sarcosyl, pH 9.5) (12).

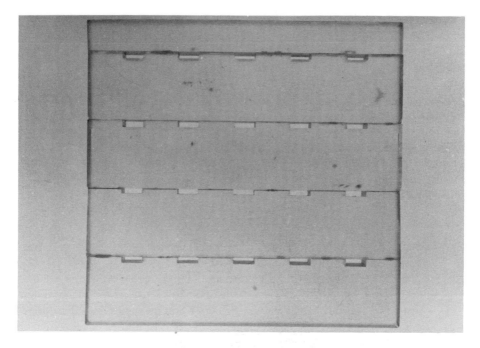

Figure 1. Perspex block mould made of 10 mm thick Perspex strips, in which 6 mm wide and 1.5 mm deep slits were made. Subsequently several strips were glued together to form the block slots.

(vii) Add proteinase K to 0.5 mg/ml, followed by 30 min incubation at room temperature and overnight incubation at 55°C. [In a later stage we have replaced the proteinase K with pronase (1-h pre-incubated) at the same concentration, followed by overnight incubation at room temperature, without noticeable effect on the results.]

(viii) Rinse the blocks several times with distilled water and wash at least three times for 2 h and once overnight in 10−20 volumes of 0.5 TE (10 mM Tris, 0.5 mM EDTA, pH 7.4), by gentle rotation.

(ix) Store the blocks at 4°C in 0.5 TE.

In our initial experiments 0.1 mM phenylmethylsulphonyl fluoride (PMSF) was added to all buffers after protease/pronase digestion (16), to block protease activity. This was later limited to the first 1−2 washes after the protease incubation.

2.2 Preparation of agarose blocks containing lambda oligomers

(i) Dilute a solution of lambda DNA of good quality (see below) to 20 μg/ml in SE, mix very gently 1:1 with 1% LMT agarose in SE at 45°C and gently dispense in slots and allow to solidify, following the procedures mentioned above.

(ii) Collect the blocks in ES, incubate for 3−5 h at 37°C and overnight at room temperature to allow annealing of the lambda sticky ends (16).

(iii) Wash the blocks and store in 0.5 TE as described above.

Various sources of lambda DNA were tested for their capacity to produce oligomers.

Commercial preparations gave variable results. Freeze-dried and frozen batches performed poorly, while preparations which had only been stored refrigerated, produced similar results as never-frozen, 'home-made' preparations. Lambda DNA preparations which had been stored refrigerated for extended periods ($>1-2$ weeks) in concentrations over 0.1 mg/ml were found to contain mainly oligomers of $200-600$ kb. The handling of these solutions needs great care (gentle pipetting, swirling in wide test tubes for mixing) to avoid shear.

A recent improvement by Smith and Cantor (Columbia University, New York), involves direct inclusion of lambda phage particles into agarose blocks at a DNA concentration of $5-10$ μg/ml, proteinase K (or pronase) treatment, followed by annealing, e.g. as described above for pure lambda DNA. This was found to yield excellent oligomeric ladders up to approximately 1.5 Mbp.

2.3 Preparation of agarose blocks containing yeast DNA

(i)   Grow haploid yeast strain YT 6.2 IL overnight in YPD to early stationary phase, dilute 1:10 and grow to a density of 1.0 OD.

(ii)   Collect the cells by centrifugation (5 min, 3000 g), resuspend in four volumes of SE, mix 1:1 with 1% LGT agarose in SE at 50°C, containing 20 mM dithiothreitol (DTT), 10 μg/ml Zymolyase 60.000 (Kyrin Breweries, Japan, or Miles).

(iii)   Pour the mixture into the block mould, chill, transfer it to an equal volume of SE$-$DTT$-$Zymolyase and incubate for 1.5 h at 37°C.

(iv)   Further process the blocks as described for blocks containing human DNA.

2.4 Restriction digestion of DNA in agarose blocks

(i)   Cut the blocks (approximate volume 100 μl) in half before use.

(ii)   Equilibrate each 50 μl block for 2 h at room temperature or overnight at 4°C with 0.5 ml of the appropriate digestion buffer.

(iii)   Replace the wash by 50 μl of fresh buffer, to which 0.1 mg/ml of bovine serum albumin (BSA) (Boehringer, MB grade) has been added.

(iv)   Carry out digestions for 6 h to overnight at the specified temperature, using $10-20$ units of enzyme for 5 μg of chromosomal DNA (equivalent to 30×10^6 cells/ml starting suspension). The enzyme is usually added in two equal portions, at the beginning and halfway through the digestion time. Control incubations without enzyme showed that the methods used produce negligible degradation of DNA in the size range under study (<2 Mb).

(v)   After digestion either layer the blocks directly or store until use in 0.5 TE at 4°C.

2.5 PFG electrophoresis

The electrophoresis system, switching intervals and blotting are described in Section 3.

(i)   Make up gels of $13.5 \times 13.5 \times 0.5$ cm, containing 1% agarose (Sigma, type I) in 0.5 $\times$ TBE (45 mM Tris, 45 mM boric acid, 0.5 mM EDTA, pH 8.3).

(ii)   Thoroughly remove the supernatant of the blocks containing digested DNA.

(iii)   Melt the blocks for 5 min at 65°C and gently pipette into the slots, using a cut-off yellow tip (suggestion of M.M.Davis, Stanford University).

(iv)   Transfer the blocks containing marker DNAs to slots pre-filled with buffer, using a Pasteur pipette bent into a hairpin and a scalpel blade.

(v)   Fix the blocks with agarose.

(vi)   Equilibrate the gel with the running buffer in the gel tray for 30−60 min. Electrophoresis is for 14−18 h at 300 V in 0.5 × TBE at various temperatures.

(viii) After electrophoresis, stain the gels for 0.5 h in 2 μg/ml ethidium bromide and de-stain for 3 h to overnight in water.

3. ELECTROPHORESIS AND BLOTTING

3.1 Sample preparation

Essentially, two methods have been described to prepare DNA of sufficient double-stranded length. We have mainly used the method described by Schwarz and Cantor (12) of including cells in agarose blocks, using the mould shown in *Figure 1*. The blocks are easy to manipulate (no centrifugations, no 'void volume' in buffer changes) and do not require increased quantities of enzymes. The alternative method is to include the cells in agarose beads by making a suspension of the still molten agarose in liquid paraffin and washing the mixture with buffer when the agarose has solidified (17). Centrifugation makes the beads settle and further treatments are essentially identical to those applied for the blocks. Both methods produce similar results in our hands in terms of the size of DNA ($\geqslant$2 Mb) and quantity of enzyme required. Choosing either method is a matter of preference, although we have consistently observed lower yields with the beads, probably due to loss of smaller particles and cells at the surface of the beads. The beads should need shorter equilibration times but, apparently, the incubation times used for the blocks allow for equilibration of buffers and enzymes.

3.2 Gel box

The electrophoresis system, cooling coil and electrical switching device are essentially as described by Carle and Olson (13). The capacity/size ratio of the box was improved to contain a larger gel (13.5 × 13.5 cm) in a smaller housing. The gel rests on a table, contained within four sets of pegs (see *Figure 2*). This method of containing the gel allows gels to be run without a supporting glass plate and allows more gels to be stacked on top of each other. Finally, two removable bars separate the open buffer inlet and outlet spaces from the main 30 × 30 cm chamber. A series of holes in each bar provides optimal cooling by guiding an even buffer stream just over the gel table.

3.3 Electrode configuration

After testing several modifications of the electrode configuration used by Carle and Olson, two improvements were included in the final design. First, the shielding of the inward 3 cm of the top electrodes (using a piece of rubber tubing, see *Figure 2C*) was found to have a profound influence on the pattern. *Figure 3* shows the separation of yeast chromosomes, lambda oligomers (*Figure 3A*) and trypanosome chromosomes (*Figure 3B*), under identical conditions, but without (*Figure 3A*) and with (*Figure 3B*) shielding. With the shielding the separation pattern becomes much straighter and a larger portion of the gel effectively contributes to the separation. Second, the bottom electrodes were put upright near the sides of the box, at the level of the bottom of the gel (*Figure 2A,B*), to provide a more convergent field. The final design of the box is shown in *Figure 2A*, a perspective drawing in *Figure 2B* and a photograph of the actual box in *Figure 2C*. The two devices visible in *Figure 2C* on the sides of the box are not essential. They were used in some stages to change the bottom electrode position. The electrode position shown in the drawings is optimal.

3.4 **Passive electrode effect**

When one electrode set is active the long passive cathode locally short-circuits the buffer along its length, accepting electrons (i.e. working as anode) near the active cathode, and releasing them (acting as cathode) near the active anode. This effect can be seen

a

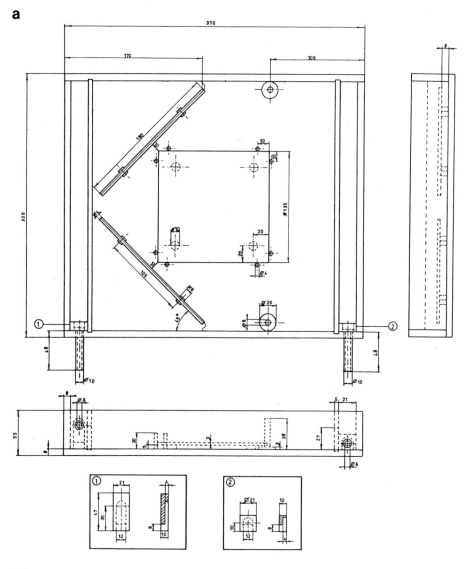

b

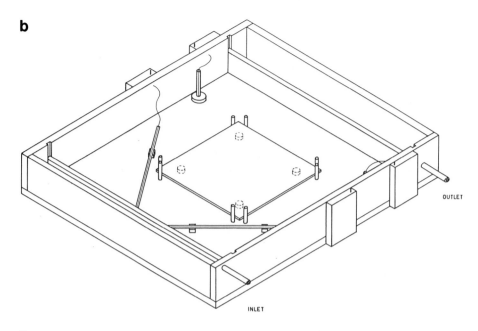

OUTLET

INLET

c

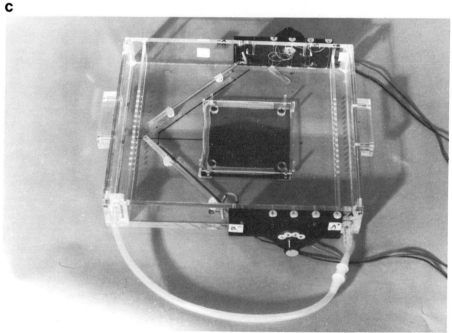

Figure 2. Panel A: line drawing of gel box and several details. **Panel B:** perspective drawing of the box. **Panel C:** photograph of the box. Note the rubber tubing to shield the inner tips of the cathodes (see text). The final position of the anodes is shown in **panels A** and **B**.

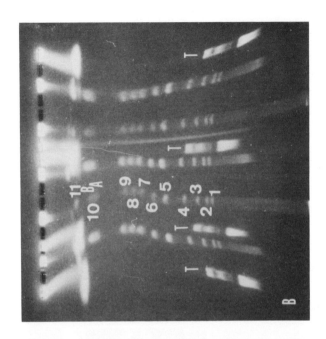

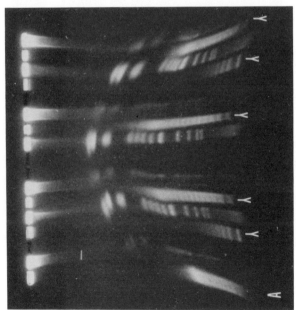

Figure 3. Effect of shielding the inner tips of the cathodes. **A:** without shielding, **B:** with shielding. Both runs are at 21°C, for 16 h at 60 sec switch time. Yeast chromosome band numbering is according to Carle and Olson (24). For chromosome length see *Table 1*.

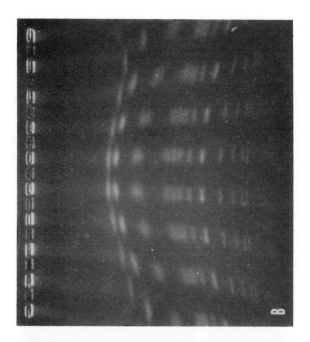

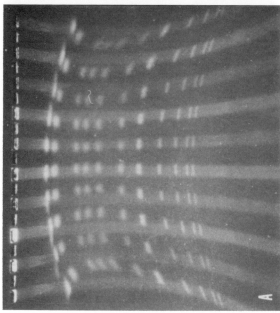

Figure 4. Difference between continuous cathode (**A**) and diode-interrupted cathode (**B**) (see text), positioned identically and using identical electrophoresis conditions (21°C, switch time 60 sec, 18 h).

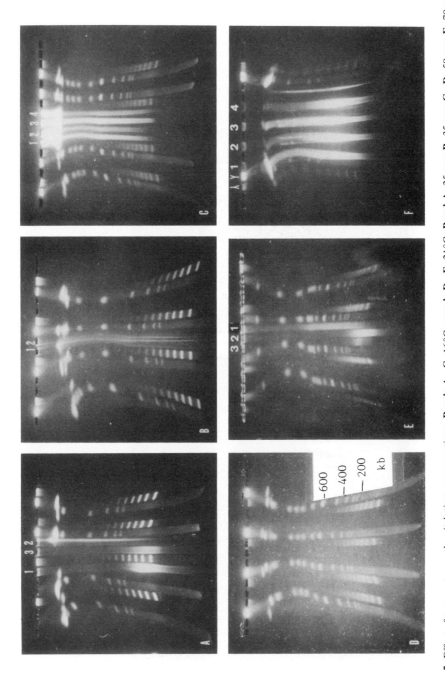

Figure 5. Effect of temperature and switch time on separations. **Panels A–C**, 16°C; **panels D–F**, 21°C. **Panel A**, 25 sec; **B**, 35 sec; **C–D**, 50 sec; **E**, 70 sec; **F**, 17 sec. All runs except **B** (18 h) lasted 14–16 h. Besides lambda oligomer ladders and yeast chromosomes, mammalian DNAs were run; see text for specific details.

during the run, by gas development on the passive cathode. Several designs are in use to prevent this effect, based upon the segmentation of the long electrode in vertical wire electrodes, interconnected by diodes to block the current in the short-circuiting direction. *Figure 4A* shows the result obtained with our standard design and *Figure 4B* that with cathodes of identical length and position, but segmented by diodes into 15 vertical wire electrodes. The latter produces a fan-shaped pattern and, although yielding sharper bands lower in the gel, it does not make optimal use of the gel surface available for resolution and allows fewer samples to be run because the side samples run off the gel. Therefore we prefer the use of a single long electrode.

3.5 Effect of switch time and temperature on separation

Figure 5 shows the dependence of the separation on the switch interval and the temperature. Panels A−C show separations at 16°C, using 25, 35 and 50 sec switch times, respectively. In these and following separations, a 'compression' zone of anomalous electrophoretic behaviour is observed, in which chromosomes of different sizes line up adjacent to each other in a fashion mirrored around the centre of the gel (cf. *Figure 3B*). In *Figure 5A* the unresolved doublet of chromosomes V and VIII (600 kb) has just left the compression region, in *Figure 5B* a triplet of approximately 820−920 kb and in *Figure 5C* an unresolved doublet of approximately 1 Mb (cf. band 10A+B in *Figure 3B*) have just left this region. A subsequent increase in running temperature from 16°C to 21°C leads to a further separation (*Figure 5D*), so this has an effect similar to increasing the switching time. A further increase in the switching time gives resolution in a still longer size range (*Figure 5E*). As can be seen in all panels, the separation of lambda oligomers is essentially linear. Comparison of the yeast patterns of the subsequent panels shows that in the top half of the gel the separation is actually extended. (The sizes mentioned above are partly derived from calibration experiments, not shown.) For chromosome allocations see Section 4.

3.6 Chromosomal DNA

Some panels of *Figure 5* also show human chromosomal DNA samples: panel A, lanes 1, 2 and 3, respectively, shows somewhat degraded DNA (20−180 kb), high molecular weight DNA, prepared by our standard protocol (10), and *Xho*I-digested DNA of lane 2. Panel B, lanes 1 and 2 shows two other samples of input high molecular weight DNA. Panel C, lanes 1−4 shows *Sal*I-digestions of human DNA samples in agarose blocks, using 10 μg (1,3) and 5 μg (2,4) of DNA per 50 μl block and 20 U of enzyme in a 6 h digestion. *Figure 5E*, lane 1 shows the DNA of *Figure 5A*, lane 2 with different switch conditions, lane 2 shows partial *Mbo*I-digested DNA of lane 1, and lane 3 the 150-kb fraction of lane 2, size-selected through a 5−25% sucrose gradient. *Figure 5F* shows *Xho*I- and *Mlu*I-digested chromosomal DNA (see legends), run at 17 sec switch time and 21°C. The blot hybridization results of *Figure 5F* are shown in *Figure 6* (see below).

From the results with the DNA in solution, we conclude that it is in principle feasible to prepare very high molecular weight DNA in solution and to carry out partial and complete digestions yielding DNA of 100−400 kb in size. This DNA can be fractionated using standard techniques. This may be practical for preparative purposes, for example

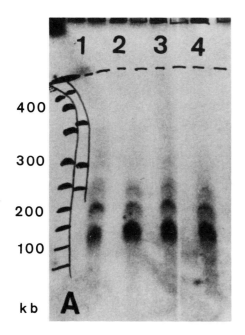
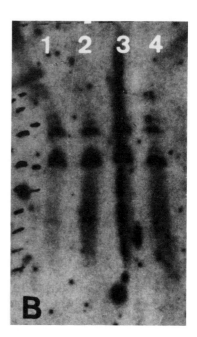

Figure 6. Blot hybridization to *Xho*I- and *Mlu*I-digested DNA. The gel shown in *Figure 5F* was blotted and hybridized with X-chromosomal probes 754 **(A)** and cX5.4 **(B)**. Digestions of 5 µg DNA: **lanes 1−2**, 10 U *Xho*I; **lane 3**, 20 U *Xho*I; **lane 4**, 40 U *Xho*I, all digestions overnight, and subsequently: **lane 2**, 2 × 10 U *Mlu*I, each for 3 h; **lane 3**, 20 U *Mlu*I, 6 h; **lane 4**, 40 U *Mlu*I, 6 h. The position of the marker lambda oligomers (outer left lane) and yeast chromosomes (inner left lane) is indicated.

re-ligation of large circles in the preparation of DNA 'jumping libraries' (18). However, great care needs to be taken to avoid shear (cut-off pipette tips, gentle mixing, preferably overnight dissolving of samples). Further, part of the size decrease in, for example, the *Xho*I digest (*Figure 5A*, lane 3) is probably due to degradation, as *Xho*I digestion of DNA in agarose leaves material greater than 600 kb (*Figure 5F*, lane 1). Obviously, when enzymes are used which cut very infrequently, like *Sal*I, where most of the digested DNA remains greater than 1 Mb (*Figure 5C*, lanes 1−4), there is no alternative to agarose-embedded DNA.

3.7 **Blotting of digested DNA**

The blotting of mammalian DNA for hybridization with single-copy probes requires efficient DNA transfer. In our hands, acid depurination gave variable results and poor sensitivity. In the course of our experiments, we have obtained good results by drying the gels (19) and hybridizing these with labelled SP6 RNA probes (B.Wieringa, University of Nijmegen, The Netherlands). However, the most convenient method of reducing the DNA size and obtaining a complete transfer by conventional blotting, is by u.v.-irradiating the ethidium bromide-stained gels, either for 40−60 sec with 254 nm light or 5 min with 302 nm light.

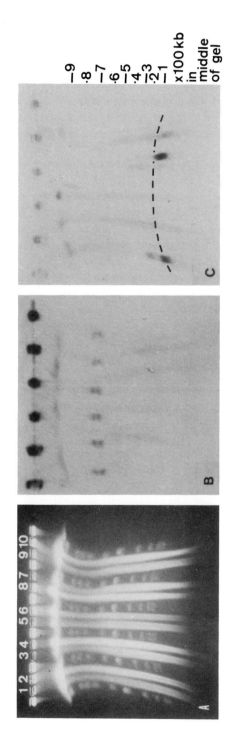

Figure 7. Digestion of human male DNA (**lanes 1,3,5,7,9**) and mouse – human hybrid DNA (**2,4,6,8,10**) with *Mlu*I (**1,2**), *Nae*I (**3,4**), *Nru*I (**5,6**), *Sst*II (**7,8**) and *Sma*I (**9,10**), using 20 units (2 × 10) to 5 µg of DNA for a 6 – 8 h digestion. Electrophoresis was at 21°C for 16 h, with 50 sec switch time. **Panel A**, gel pattern; **B**, hybridization with probe 754; **C**, hybridization with human ADA cDNA probe. For the length of the yeast chromosomes see *Table 1*. The bands in **panel C** are (**lane 1**) 320 and 430 kb, (**lane 7**) 280 kb.

3.8 **Results using unique probes**

Figure 5F shows an *Xho*I and *Mlu*I digestion of normal female DNA and *Figure 6A* the blot hybridization with the human X-chromosomal probe 754. Lanes 1 and 2 contain DNA digested with 10 U of *Xho*I, lanes 3 and 4 with 20 and 40 U of *Xho*I. The DNA of lanes 2−4 was subsequently digested with various amounts of *Mlu*I: twice with 10 U for 3 h (lane 2), once with 20 U (lane 3) and once with 40 U (lane 4). *Figure 5F* shows that *Mlu* digestion reduces the amount of *Xho*I-digested DNA left in the compression region and that above approximately 300 kb. The hybridization patterns are nearly identical, however, with the exception of minor bands higher in the gel. Since the probe does not contain an *Xho*I site, the multiple bands indicate incomplete digestion. Since overdigestion has no effect, this is probably due to partial resistance of the sites to cleavage (see Section 5.3). The major *Xho*I fragments detected are 130 and 200 kb long.

Figure 7A shows digestion of human male (odd lanes) and mouse−human hybrid DNA (even lanes). The hybrid line contains only the Xp21-proximal segment of the human X-chromosome. The digestions are with *Mlu*I (lanes 1,2), *Nae*I (lanes 3,4), *Nru*I (lanes 5,6), *Sst*II (lanes 7,8, note that the lanes are inverted) and *Sma*I (lanes 9,10). *Figure 7B* shows the hybridization of this blot to the X-probe 754 and *Figure 7C* to an adenosine deaminase (ADA) cDNA probe (20). The latter gene maps to chromosome 20 (21). The strong hybridization in *Figure 7B* to the slots and the doublet band at one-third of the gel are due to contamination of the yeast blocks used with plasmid-containing *Escherichia coli* and are not relevant. Probe 754 does not show specific bands. The ADA probe (excised from its plasmid) produces specific bands with *Mlu*I- and *Sst*II-digested human DNA (lanes 1,7) of 320 and 420 kb (lane 1) and 280 kb (lane 7, note the curvature of the markers) and a weak signal with the mouse homologue in the *Sst*II lane (lane 8). In the other lanes no bands are discernible. The other enzymes used thus may have no accessible sites in the vicinity of the probes. For probe 754 with the *Mlu*I digest this is at least consistent with the double digestion results with *Xho*I in *Figure 7*. Finally, *Figure 8* shows the hybridization of 754 to *Sfi*I-digested normal female DNA (lane 1) and DNA of a glycerol kinase patient deleted for 754 (14) (lane 2). Here a single fragment of 850 kb is clearly detected, which is missing from the deleted DNA.

Another Xp21-probe, cX5.4, which lies within 1−2 Mb centromeric of 754 (22), detects *Xho*I fragments of 300 and 350 kb (*Figure 6C*), with minor bands at 310, 360 and 370 kb. Additional digestions are required to construct a map for both regions and to determine, if possible, the distance between the two Xp21 probes.

4. YEAST CHROMOSOMES AS A MARKER SYSTEM

Since the first demonstration by Schwarz *et al.* (23), that very large DNA molecules could be separated on agarose gels, essentially by forcing them to reorientate continuously in the gel matrix, the technique of PFG electrophoresis (12), or orthogonal field alternation gel electrophoresis (OFAGE) (13) has been effectively used for the electrophoretic chromosome separation of primitive eukaryotes such as yeast (12,13,24), trypanosomes (25) and *Plasmodium* (26). Only recently has the technique been combined with the use of restriction enzymes to study trypanosome DNA (16). For the application of the

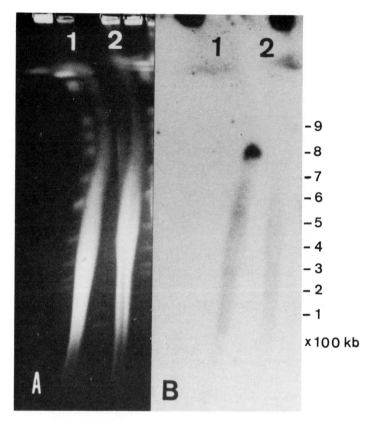

Figure 8. *Sfi*I digestion **(A)** and hybridization **(B)** of probe 754 to human female DNA **(lanes 1)** and DNA of a male glycerol kinase-deficient patient deleted for a region around the 754 locus (14) **(lanes 2)**.

system to restriction analysis of mammalian (human) DNA, in a size range of 50−2000 kb, the yeast chromosomes serve as a very useful marker system.

The fractionation pattern we obtain for the yeast chromosomes corresponds to that obtained by Carle and Olson (24). We have numbered the bands in *Figure 3B* according to their nomenclature and *Table 1* shows the lengths we find for the chromosomes in bands 1−9, using lambda DNA oligomers for calibration in the presented and additional experiments. The chromosomal sizes reported by Carle and Olson correspond very well with our data. Their data set has been obtained at 50 sec switching time, when we find 260 kb and 300 kb for bands 1 and 2 (*Figure 5C*), compared with 260 and 290 kb found by them. At shorter switch times, which give a better resolution in this region, lengths of 240 and 280 kb are obtained (*Figures 5A* and *B*). The calibration differences are less than 20 kb. We find that the migration behaviour of the yeast chromosomes relative to the lambda oligomers is highly reproducible. Bands 10A and 10B are sometimes better separated than at other times (cf. *Figures 3B* and *5A−E*). It has yet to be established, however, whether mammalian DNAs also migrate in this almost condition-independent manner.

Table 1. Size fractionation of yeast chromosomes.

Band no.	Chromosome(s)	Length (kb)
12	IV	
11	VII, XV	
10B	XVI	
10A	XIII	
9	II	920
8	XIV	870
7	X	820
6	XI	710
5	V, VIII	600
4	IX	450
3	III	350
2	VI	290
1	I	250

Band nomenclature and chromosome allocation is according to Carle and Olson (24). Sizes are calibrated with commercially available lambda CI857Sam7 variant (49 kb) and show a ± 10 kb spreading between runs with different switching times (see text).

5. RESTRICTION ANALYSIS OF MAMMALIAN DNA

5.1 Resolution

A very important feature of the PFG technique is the near linearity of the separation. This produces an excellent resolution, which actually increases higher in the gel. In principle, therefore, length differences of 10−20 kb are detected with equal ease in fragments ranging in size from 100 to 800 kb. This makes the technique very powerful for the detection of minor deletions or rearrangements at great distances from the probes used.

5.2 Enzyme selection

Given the separation range of the PFG system, restriction enzymes have to be selected which cleave very infrequently. The enzymes having found the widest application thus far, recognize hexanucleotides or smaller sequences, producing fragments of, on average, a few kilobases and ranging from 10 bp up to approximately 50 kb. Only a few commercially available enzymes recognize octameric or longer sequences, notably *Not*I (GCGGCCGC) and *Sfi*I (GGCCNNNNNGGCC). In addition, enzymes may be chosen with one or more CpG dinucleotides in their recognition site, as these sequences are under-represented in the genome by one order of magnitude (27). *Table 2* lists most of these enzymes and their recognition sequences. Additional specificities may be generated by judicious combination of restriction endonucleases and methylases (see, for example, N.E.Biolabs Catalogue 1985/1986). This approach has already been applied to agarose-embedded DNA (16).

As expected, DNA cleaved with the enzymes of *Table 2* shows a digestion smear of 50−2000 kb (*Figures 5−8*). However, the combined use of CpG-specific enzymes and unique probes for the short arm of the X-chromosome yields incomplete digestion with *Xho*I (*Figure 6*) and no discrete hybridization at all with *Mlu*I, *Nar*I, *Nru*I, *Sst*II

Table 2. Restriction enzymes which cleave infrequently in mammalian DNA.

*Asu*II	TTCGAA		
*Aat*II	GACGTC	*Pae*R7I	CTCGAG
*Bss*HII	CGCGCG	*Pvu*I	CGATCG
*Cla*I	ATCGAT	*Sac*II (*Sst*II)	CCGCGG
*Fsp*I	TGCGCA	*Sal*I	GTCGAC
*Mlu*I	ACGCGT	*Sfi*I	GGCCNNNNNGGCC
*Nae*I	GCCGGC	*Sma*I (*Xma*I)	CCCGGG
*Nar*I	GGCGCC	*Sna*BI	TACGTA
*Not*I	GCGGCCGC	*Xho*I	CTCGAG
*Nru*I	TCGCGA	*Xma*III	CGGCCG

and *Sma*I (*Figure 7B*). The latter result could either imply the total absence of sites in the wide surroundings of the probes, or a yet more incomplete digestion. Control hybridization of the blot of *Figure 7A* with an ADA cDNA probe (20), which maps to chromosome 20 (21) (*Figure 7C*), shows identifiable bands with *Mlu*I at 320 and 420 kb and with *Sst*II at 280 kb (note the curvature of the calibration), while a similar lack of specific cleavage is seen with the other enzymes. This strongly suggests that the digestion is essentially complete and that the results depend on the combination of enzyme and probe used. The ADA hybridization is specific, since the adjacent mouse DNA lanes are highlighted only very faintly with the ADA cDNA probe.

5.3 Methylation

We have varied the amount of several enzymes (e.g. *Xho*I, *Mlu*I, *Sal*I, *Sfi*I) from 1 to 8 U/μg of DNA, added twice during a 6 h digestion period without noticeable effect on either digestion or hybridization pattern. First this shows that digestion of agarose-embedded DNA requires conditions similar to soluble digestion, and second it implies once more that the observed underdigestion has a more fundamental reason, probably related to the CpG dinucleotide being the main target for methylation in mammalian DNA. In fact, methylation and under-representation of CpG in the genome are causally related (28) and methylation and inactivation are closely linked (29). The most likely explanation for the results is partial methylation of the sites studied. Consistent with its site lacking CpG, *Sfi*I gives complete digestion (*Figure 8*). *Sfi*I may thus become pivotal in this type of analysis.

The possibility that female X-inactivation plays a major part in the putative methylation as a cause for incomplete digestion, is unlikely. The human DNA of *Figure 7* is of male origin and the autosomal ADA probe shows a similar effect with some of the enzymes. Inactivation may however produce methylation differences in other X-chromosomal regions and PFG electrophoresis may become another useful tool in the study of X-inactivation.

5.4 GC-cluster mapping

An interesting approach to the digestion problem has been followed by W.Brown and A.Bird (Edinburgh). The promoter sequences for several so-called 'household genes', such as HMG-CoA reductase (30), hypoxanthine phosphoribosyl transferase (HPRT)

(31) and ADA (20), which are constitutively expressed, lack a TATA-box but contain very GC-rich sequences (32). In these regions, the CpG dinucleotide is not under-represented, probably because these sequences belong to constitutively active regions and are thus rarely if ever methylated. These GC-rich sequences usually contain sites for one or more of the enzymes of *Table 2*. By screening random cosmid clones for the presence of clustered sites for these enzymes, and subsequently isolating unique subclones adjacent to these clusters, Brown and co-workers have been able to construct restriction maps of regions of 200−400 kb around the dihydrofolate reductase (DHFR) gene and two random GC-rich sequences. They found that in most cases studied, the sites distal to the probes also tended to cluster and that, in the regions under study, these site clusters map 60−200 kb apart. The experiment of *Figure 7C* with the ADA probe yields similar results with *Mlu*I and *Sst*II. However, as only about 5% of the random cosmids contained site clusters, their average spacing throughout the genome may be quite variable. Our observations with the Xp21-specific probes show that in this particular region unmethylated GC-clusters are scarce, if present at all.

6. PFG ELECTROPHORESIS: THEORETICAL MODELS

Although several practical designs for the PFG electrophoresis system have been shown to work (12,13), the exact basis of the separation is still open to much speculation. A general observation is that both open circular and supercoiled molecules migrate anom-alously slowly in this system (12,24), suggesting that linear molecules are not extensively coiled during their movement. Theoretically, the retarded migration of an open circle implies that the presence of as little as two hairpin folds in a molecule is already capable of slowing it down relative to its linear equivalent. Another general observation is that the resolution increases when the field angle becomes wider. This is also the net effect obtained by our shielding of the inward ends of the cathodes.

These observations have led Southern (University of Oxford) to propose (EMBL meet-ing on Approaches to Genome Analysis, October 1985) that the DNA strands, after migrating with equal velocity during a switch cycle as strings or rods of different lengths, are separated by being pulled away from their tails in the other direction. Molecules of different sizes, starting simultaneously, will end one cycle with their tails at a dif-ferent position, the longest having its tail closest to the starting position. When these tails migrate first in the sideways direction, a net separation will result, with the longer molecule migrating closer to the original start position. This resolution will gradually increase during the run. As Southern points out, his model explains both the linear relationship between size and mobility and the fact that field angles less than 90° are unfavourable, since this allows the original head to 'round the corner' and hence does not increase separation.

Strikingly however, Olson (Washington University, St. Louis) demonstrated at the same meeting (G.R.Carle and M.V.Olson, manuscript submitted) that separation is also obtained by switching the polarity back and forth in a classical horizontal gel appar-atus, with frequencies ranging from 0.25 to 60 sec, with the 'forward' cycle having longer periods than the 'backward' cycle. This is an important advancement of the tech-nique, since it yields straight bands. Olson explains the results by proposing that during migration of the molecules, whatever their precise shape, they acquire a non-identical 'head' and 'tail' (e.g. a wedge shape). When the polarity is inverted, the molecules have to reorganize themselves before being able to move in the new direction. The time this takes depends on the molecular size, hence the net resolution obtained when this process is continuously repeated, with a longer forward cycle to yield net motion.

At face value, these observations contradict Southern's model, since that seems to require an angle between the fields. However, both models place emphasis on non-identity of heads and tails. We propose the following adaptation, reconciling both models and explaining most of the observations thus far. When a large random coil starts to be pulled through a fine grid, it will try to enter at many positions along its length. Net motion is only achieved after one of the random bends (or kinks) has 'won', unfolding all the other bends and producing a hairpin-folded, V-shaped molecule. This will clearly have properties consistent with the Olson-model: inverting the polarity causes the molecule to get stuck until a new head has developed. The Southern model equally applies when it is not based upon the tail position but on the average position of every molecule. It will be from this average position that a new hairpin-head will usually be formed and pulled away sideways when the field direction is switched. The hairpin model explains, in a similar fashion to Southern's model, why field angles over 90° are favourable.

7. FUTURE APPLICATIONS

PFG electrophoresis is a powerful new technique, equally promising for the analysis of the genomes of prokaryotes, primitive eukaryotes and mammals. The impact of incomplete digestion remains to be evaluated. We have evidence that this problem may be partly overcome by the use of transformed cell lines, as these consistently produce more completely digested patterns than, for example, lymphoid cells. In some specific cases the use of tissue in which the region of interest is expressed and hence under-methylated will be possible. On the other hand, partial digestion by itself extends the detection range of restriction sites, thus permitting the mapping of several adjacent sites, provided the pattern does not become too complex. Direct control of the digestion of rare recognition sites can be obtained by hybridization of probes from their immediate vicinity to a double digest with a frequently cutting enzyme, electrophoresed on a conventional gel, verifying double digestion of the fragment produced with the second enzyme alone (W.Brown, Edinburgh). The specific cloning of probes adjacent to rare sites, by double digestion of genomic DNA with the particular enzyme and, for example, *Eco*RI or *Bam*HI, followed by shotgun cloning in a vector with compatible ends, as applied by C.Smith (Columbia University, New York) for the construction of a restriction map of the *E. coli* genome, provides an interesting means of constructing and linking up maps of large, adjacent genomic regions.

Finally, the development of a conventional, horizontal electrophoresis technique with similar resolution properties using the field inversion-technique (33) will be of great practical value for routine preparative and diagnostic applications of the technique. The rare hexamer-cutting enzymes can be predicted to have an increased RFLP frequency, due to their sites containing the mutation-sensitive CpG sequence, like *Taq*I and *Msp*I amongst the tetramer cutters. Thus, applications of the technique can be envisaged not only in physical linkage studies as shown above but also in genetic linkage analysis.

But even with the current state of the technique, there is no reason to delay its introduction into the laboratory. The equipment as shown, including the switching device (13), can be made by any skilled workshop and a standard power supply capable of providing 300 V and 200 mA is sufficient to perform the separations.

8. ACKNOWLEDGEMENTS

We gratefully acknowledge the kind and skilful assistance of C.R.G.van der Geest, R.D.Runia and L.Gerrese in the construction and adaptations of the PFG box and electronic equipment, Mrs E.Klein-Breteler for technical assistance in tissue culture, Dr O.Myklebost for collaboration, Mr A.Van der Bliek and Dr A.Bernards for helpful discussions, Dr A.Bernards for gifts of trypanosome samples, Mrs A.Kempers for gifts of yeast samples and strains, Dr D.Valerio for a gift of ADA cDNA, Professor P.L. Pearson for critically reading the manuscript and Professor P.Borst for his hospitality in the initial phase of our work. This work was performed with the financial aid of the Netherlands Prevention Fund grant no. 28.878.

9. REFERENCES

1. van Ommen,G.J.B., Arnberg,A.C., Baas,F., Brocas,H., Sterk,A., Tegelaers,W.H.H., Vassart,G. and de Vÿlder,J.J.M. (1983) *Nucleic Acids Res.*, **11**, 2273.
2. Baas,F., Bikker,H., Geurts van Kessel,A., Melsert,R., Pearson,P.L., de Vÿlder,J.J.M. and van Ommen, G.J.B. (1985) *Hum. Genet.*, **69**, 138.
3. Steinmetz,M., Winoto,A., Minard,K. and Hood,L. (1982) *Cell*, **28**, 489.
4. Weiss,E.H., Golden,L., Fahrner,K., Mellor,A.L., Devlin,J.J., Bullman,H., Tiddens,H., Bud,H. and Flavell,R.A. (1984) *Nature*, **310**, 650.
5. Kedes,L.H. (1985) *Trends Genet.*, **1**, 205.
6. Davies,K.E., Pearson,P.L., Harper,P.S., Murray,J.M., O'Brien,T.O., Sartarazi,M. and Williamson,R. (1983) *Nucleic Acids Res.*, **11**, 2302.
7. Emery,A.E.H. (1983) in *Principles and Practice of Medical Genetics*, Emery,A.E.H. and Rimoin,D.L. (eds), Churchill-Livingston, London, p.392.
8. Pembrey,M.E. (1982) *Am. J. Med. Genet.*, **12**, 437.
9. Verellen-Dumoulin,Ch., Freund,M., Demeyer,R., Laterre,Ch., Frédéric,J., Thompson,M.W., Markovic,V.D. and Worton,R.C. (1984) *Hum. Genet.*, **67**, 115−119.
10. Hofker,M.H., Wapenaar,M.C., Goor,N., Bakker,E., van Ommen,G.J.B. and Pearson,P.L. (1985) *Hum. Genet.*, **70**, 148.
11. Francke,U., Ochs,H.D., de Martinville,B., Giacalore,J., Lindgren,V., Disteche,C., Pagon,R.A., Hofker,M.H., van Ommen,G.J.B., Pearson,P.L. and Wedgwood,R. (1985) *Am. J. Hum. Genet.*, **67**, 250.
12. Schwarz,D.C. and Cantor,C.R. (1984) *Cell*, **37**, 67.
13. Carle,G.F. and Olson,M.V. (1984) *Nucleic Acids Res.*, **12**, 5647.
14. Wieringa,B., Hustinx,Th., Scheres,J., Renier,W., Ter Haar,B. (1985) *Clin. Genet.*, **27**, 522.
15. Monaco,A.P., Bertelson,C.J., Middlesworth,W., Colleti,C.-A., Aldridge,J., Fishbeck,K.H., Bartlett,R., Pericak-Vance,M.A., Roses,A.D. and Kunkel,L.M. (1985) *Nature*, **316**, 842.
16. Bernards,A., Kooter,J.M., Michels,P.A.M., Moberts,R.M.P. and Borst,P. (1986) *Gene*, in press.
17. Jackson,D.A. and Cook,P.R. (1985) *EMBO J.*, **4**, 913.
18. Collins,F.J. and Weissman,S.M. (1984) *Proc. Natl. Acad. Sci. USA*, **81**, 6812.
19. Studencki,A.B. and Wallace,R. (1984) *DNA*, **3**, 7.
20. Valerio,D., Duyvesteyn,M.G.C., Dekker,B.M.M., Weeda,G., Berkvens,Th.M., Van der Voorn,L., van Ormondt,H. and Van der Eb,A.J. (1985) *EMBO J.*, **4**, 437.
21. Valerio,D., Duyvesteyn,M.G.C., Meera Khan,P., Geurts van Kessel,A., de Waard,A. and van der Eb,A.J. (1983) *Gene*, **25**, 231.
22. van Ommen,G.J.B., Bakker,E., Hofker,M.H., Skraastad,M., Bergen,A., Goor,N., Sandkuyl,L., van Essen,W.J. and Pearson,P.L. (1985) in *Biotechnology in Diagnostics*, Koprowski,H., Ferrone,S. and Albertini,A. (eds.), Elsevier, Amsterdam, p. 255.

23. Schwartz,D.C., Saffran,W., Welsh,J., Haas,R., Goldenberg,M. and Cantor,C.R. (1982) *Cold Spring Harbor Symp. Quant. Biol.*, **47**, 189.
24. Carle,G.F. and Olson,M.V. (1985) *Proc. Natl. Acad. Sci. USA*, **82**, 3756.
25. Van der Ploeg,L.H.T., Schwartz,D.C., Cantor,C.R. and Borst,P. (1984) *Cell*, **37**, 77.
26. Kemp,D.J., Corcoran,L.M., Coppel,R.L., Stahl,H.D., Bianco,A.E., Brown,G.V. and Anders,R.F. (1985) *Nature*, **315**, 347.
27. Bird,A.P. (1980) *Nucleic Acids Res.*, **8**, 1499.
28. Coulondre,C., Miller,J.H., Farabaugh,P.J. and Gilbert,W. (1978) *Nature*, **274**, 755.
29. Shen,C.-K.J. and Maniatis,T. (1980) *Proc. Natl. Acad. Sci. USA*, **77**, 6634.
30. Reynolds,G.A., Basu,S.K., Osborne,T.F., Chin,D.J., Gil,G., Brown,M.S., Goldstein,J.L. and Luskey,K.L. (1984) *Cell*, **38**, 275.
31. Melton,D.W., Konecki,D.S., Brennand,J. and Caskey,C.T. (1984) *Proc. Natl. Acad. Sci. USA*, **81**, 2147.
32. Bird,A., Taggart,M., Frommer,M., Miller,O.J. and Macleod,D. (1985) *Cell*, **40**, 91.
33. Carle,G.F., Frank,M. and Olson,M.V. (1986) *Science*, **232**, 65.

Suppliers of specialist items

The following list is not intended to be exhaustive but rather to give addresses of suppliers of reagents and instruments cited in this book. Many of the larger companies have subsidiaries in other countries whilst most of the smaller companies also market their products through agents. The name of a local supplier is most easily obtained by writing to the relevant address listed here, which is usually the head office.

Amersham International plc, White Lion Road, Amersham, Buckinghamshire, HP7 9LL, UK

Anglian Biotechnology Ltd., Unit 8, Hawkins Road, Colchester, Essex CO2 8JX, UK

BDH Chemicals Ltd., Broom Road, Poole, Dorset BH12 4NN, UK

Becton Dickinson, 490B, Lakeside Drive, Sunnyvale, CA 94086, USA

Bethesda Research Laboratories Inc., P.O. Box 6009, Gaithersburg, MD 20877, USA

BioRad Laboratories Ltd., 2200 Wright Avenue, Richmond, CA 94804, USA
Also Caxton Way, Watford, Hertfordshire, UK

Boehringer Mannheim Biochemica, P.O. Box 31020, D-6800 Mannheim, FRG
Also Boehringer Mannheim House, Bell Lane, Lewes, East Sussex BN7 1LG, UK

BRL; see Bethesda Research Laboratories.

Calbiochem-Behring, La Jolla, CA 92037, USA

Cambridge Biotechnology Laboratories Ltd., Uniscience Ltd., 12-14 St. Ann's Crescent, London SW18 2LS, UK

Cambridge Life Sciences plc, Cambridge Science Park, Milton Road, Cambridge, CB4 4BH, UK

Collaborative Research Inc., 1365 Main Street, Waltham, MA 02154, USA

Difco Laboratories Ltd., P.O. Box 14B, Central Avenue, East Molesey, Surrey KT8 OSE, UK

Du Pont Instruments, Peck's Lane, Newton, CT 06470, USA

Eastman Kodak Co., 343 State Street, Rochester, NY 14650, USA

Enzo-Biochem Inc., 325 Hudson Street, New York, NY 10013, USA

Ernst Leitz Wetzler GmbH, D-6330 Wetzler, FRG

Falcon. Products available from Becton Dickinson U.K. Ltd., Between Towns Road, Cowley, Oxford OX4 3LY, UK

Fisons Chemicals Ltd., Bishop Meadow Road, Loughborough LE11 ORG, UK

Flow Laboratories Inc., 7655 Old Springhouse Road, McLean, VA 22101, USA

Fluka AG, CH-9470 Buchs, Switzerland

Fuji Photofilm Co., 26-30 Nishiazabu 2-chome, Minato-ku, Tokyo 106, Japan

Gallenkamp Co. Ltd., Technico House, Christopher Street, London, EC2P 2ER, UK

Gibco Ltd., P.O. Box 35, Trident House, Renfrew Road, Paisley PA3 4EF, UK

Gilson. Products available from Anachem Ltd., 15 Power Court, Luton, Bedfordshire LU1 3JJ, UK

Ilford, 14-22 Tottenham Street, London W1P OAH, UK

Kodak Ltd., Kodak House, Station Road, Hemel Hempstead, Hertfordshire HP1 1JU, UK

Life Sciences Inc., 2900 72nd Street North, St. Petersburg, FL 33710, USA (products available from Anglian Biotechnology Ltd. and Northumbria Biologicals Ltd. in the UK)

Merck, D-6100 Darmstadt, FRG

Miles Laboratories, P.O. Box 37, Stoke Poges, Slough SL2 4LY, UK
Also P.O. Box 2000, Elkart, IN 46515, USA

Millipore, Ashby Road, Bedford, MA 01730, USA
Also 11-15 Peterborough Road, Harrow, Middlesex, UK

New England Biolabs Inc., 32 Tozer Road, Beverley, MA 01915, USA
Also products available from CP Laboratories Ltd, P.O. Box 22, Bishops Stortford, Hertfordshire, UK

New England Nuclear, Postfach 401240, D-6072 Dreieich, FRG
Also 549 Albany Street, Boston, MA 02118, USA

NEN; see New England Nuclear.

Northumbria Biologicals Ltd, S. Nelson Industrial Estate, Cramlington, NE23 9HL, UK

Oxoid Ltd., Wade Road, Basingstoke RG24 OPW, UK

Pharmacia Fine Chemicals AB, P.O. Box 175, S-75104 Uppsala-1, Sweden.

Pierce Chemical Co., P.O. Box 117, Rockford, IL 61105, USA

P-L Biochemicals Inc., see Pharmacia Fine Chemicals AB

P and S Biochemicals, 38 Queensland Street, Liverpool L7 3JG, UK

Promega Biotech, 2800 S. Fish Hatchery Road, Madison, WI 53711, USA
Also products available from P and S Biochemicals, 38 Queensland Street, Liverpool L7 3JG, UK

Raven Scientific Ltd., Sturmer End, Haverhill, Suffolk, England

Sartorius Instruments Ltd., 18 Avenue Road, Belmont, Surrey SM2 6JD, UK

Sartorius GmbH, Postfach 19, D-3400 Göttingen, FRG

Schleicher and Schuell. Products available from Anderman & Co. Ltd., 145 London Road, Kingston-upon-Thames, Surrey KT2 6NH, UK

Sigma Chemical Co. Ltd., Fancy Road, Poole, Dorset BH17 7NH, UK
Also P.O. Box 14508, St. Louis, MO 63178, USA

Whatman Ltd., Springfield Mill, Maidstone, Kent ME14 2LE, UK

Worthington Biochemical Corporation, Freehold, NJ 07728, USA

INDEX

Agarose blocks, 114
Agarose gels, dried, 39
Ammonium acetate precipitation, 2
Amniotic fluid, 2
  DNA extraction, 4

Base pair mismatch, 34, 37
Berk and Sharp mapping, 70
Biotinylation, 61
Blotting, 7, 117
  high molecular weight DNA, 14

cDNA, 65
Cells,
  DNA extraction, 4
  lysis, 103, 104
Centimorgan, 20
Chorionic villi, 1
  DNA yield, 3
Chromogenic detection, 63
Chromosome abnormality, 107
Chromosome banding, 88, 95
Chromosome centrifugation, 101
Chromosome DNA library, 110
Chromosome preparations,
  for in situ, 86, 90
  for flow cytometry, 103
Colcemid, 102
Computer programs,
  linkage, 25
Confidence limits, 28

Denhardt's solution, 7, 78
Developing in situ slides, 93
Dextran sulphate, 36
Diazotization, 53
DNA chromosome library, 110
DNA extraction,
  villi, 2
  amniotic fluid, 3
  blood, 5, 56
  cultured cells, 4
DNA strains, 105
DNA storage, 5
DNA coupling to resin, 52
Dot blot, 68
Double back-cross, 23
Duplex stability, 33

Electrophoresis,
  agarose, 7
  PFG, 117
Electrode, 117

Emulsion, 88
5′ end labelling, 40
Enzymes,
  restriction digest, 6
  infrequent cutters, 128
Exonuclease VII, 72, 83

Fetal loss, 15
Flow cytometry, 101
Flow karotype analysis, 107
Fluorochrome, 101, 105

$G+C$ content, 37
G-C cluster mapping, 129
Gene deletion, 10
Gene frequency, 26
Gene mapping, 109
Gene order, 24
Genetic distance, 26
Genetic linkage, 19
Genetic risk, 30
Genomic DNA, 65
Genotype, 21
Grain distribution, 95

Heterogeneity (linkage), 29
Hybrid stability, 34, 87
Hybridization kinetics, 35
Hybridization,
  buffer, 7
  immobilised DNA, 57
  non-radioactive probes, 61
  Southern blots, 7
  in situ, 92

In situ hybridization, 85
  resolution, 99
Interference, 24
Interval estimates, 28
Introns, 67
Isotopes,
  in situ, 86

Karyotype,
  flow sorting, 103, 107
Kinase labelling, 54

Labelling,
  end-labelling, 40, 43
  hexanucleotide, 7
  kinase labelling, 40
  nick translation, 7, 55
  oligolabelling, 7, 55
  primer extension, 40, 43
Lambda fragments, 115